# Life, Liberty and the Defense of Dignity

## The Challenge for Bioethics

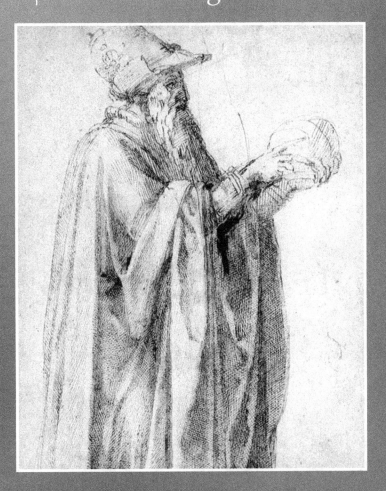

## Leon R. Kass, M.D.

# Life, Liberty and the Defense of Dignity

## The Challenge for Bioethics

Leon R. Kass M.D.

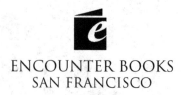

ENCOUNTER BOOKS
SAN FRANCISCO

First paperback edition published in 2004 by Encounter Books, an activity of Encounter for Culture and Education, Inc., a nonprofit tax exempt corporation.

Encounter Books website address: www.encounterbooks.com

Manufactured in the United States and printed on acid-free paper.

The paper used in this publication meets the minimum requirements of ANSI/NISO Z39.48-1992 (R 1997) (*Permanence of Paper*).

Library of Congress Cataloging-in-Publication Data

Kass, Leon.
    Life, liberty, and the defense of dignity : the challenge for bioethics /
Leon R. Kass
        p.   cm.
    Includes bibliographical references and index (p. ).
    ISBN 1-1-59403-047-2 (alk. paper)
    1. Bioethics.   I. Title.
QH332 .K37 2002
174'.957—dc21

                                                    2002074225


10  9  8  7  6  5  4  3  2  1

To three bright lights that have illuminated my journey

Harvey Flaumenhaft
*In memoriam,* Hans Jonas (1903–1993)
*In memoriam,* Paul Ramsey (1913–1988)

# Contents

# Introduction

S tem cells. Cloning. The Human Genome Project. If the year 2001 was any indication, issues of bioethics will be a dominant concern of the new century—indeed, of the new millennium. For much of the year, before the events of September 11 relegated everything else to the back page, the United States was absorbed in a difficult moral debate about whether the federal government should fund research on human embryonic stem cells. Proponents touted the lifesaving and disease-curing promise of these pluripotent cells, which may someday enable doctors to replace tissues damaged by spinal cord injury, juvenile diabetes or Parkinson's disease, among others. Opponents objected to the necessary exploitation and destruction of the human embryos from which the stem cells are extracted.

In August 2001, in his first major televised address to the nation, President Bush announced his solution. Intent on reaffirming the moral principle that nascent life not be destroyed for the sake of research, yet eager to explore the possible therapeutic benefits of these cells, he chose to permit federal funds to be used for research only on already existing embryonic stem cell lines. At the same time, he announced the creation of a President's Council on Bioethics to monitor stem cell research and to consider all of the medical and ethical ramifications of biomedical innovation. I was appointed to chair this council. The President has directed it to lead a "fundamental inquiry into the human and moral significance of developments in biomedical and behavioral science and technology." He wants everyone to understand that the stem cell question, important in its own right, is but the forerunner of a horde of similar questions that we will need to confront, sooner rather than later.

The subject of embryo research is not new, and neither is human cloning, the other hotly debated bioethical topic of the past year. Both matters surfaced in the late 1960s and 1970s, following the successful cloning of tadpoles (1962) and the birth of the first human "test-tube baby" (1978). And I am not new to these subjects. In the

1970s I published several essays on laboratory-assisted reproduction, cloning, and manipulation of human embryos,[1] the last based on testimony I had given in 1978 before a National Institutes of Health Ethics Advisory Board on the very question of federal funding of human embryo research. The questions we face today are not identical to those of twenty-five years ago. For one thing, no one then was talking about stem cells or the prospects for regenerative medicine. Yet despite changes in the science and technology, the basic moral and political questions remain the same: What does it mean to treat nascent human life as raw material to be exploited as a mere natural resource? What does it mean to blur the line between procreation and manufacture? What are the likely future technical possibilities and moral problems that our present decisions are willy-nilly creating? What moral boundaries should researchers observe, whether they work with federal or with private funds? What are the goals of, and what are the proper limits to, the project for the mastery of human nature? Can we control where this project is taking us, so as to reap the benefits without losing our humanity? If so, how?

Our recent policy debates, like so many other arguments about biomedical technology, tend to neglect these larger questions. We find ourselves reacting piecemeal and ad hoc to the latest biotechnological possibility without seeing its meaning whole. We largely ignore its contribution to the growing power for altering and controlling human bodies and minds. More important, we lack a rich enough understanding of the human goods we wish to preserve and defend. We need to realize that there is more at stake in the biological revolution than just saving life or avoiding death and suffering. We must also strive to protect and preserve human dignity and the ideas and practices that keep us human. This book is an invitation to remember these human and moral concerns, concerns that are themselves manifestations of what is humanly most worth preserving.

To place our moral inquiry in context, let us remind ourselves at the outset that 2001 was also the year in which our world was drastically changed, and with it our nation's mood and attention. In numerous if subtle ways, since September 11 there is a palpable increase in America's moral seriousness, well beyond the expected defense of our values and institutions so viciously under attack. We have rallied in support of the respect for life, liberty, the rule of law and the pursuit of progress. But we seem to have acquired in addition a deepened appreciation of human finitude and vulnerability, and therefore of the preciousness of the ties that bind and the importance of making good use of our allotted span of years. A fresh breeze of sensible moral judgment, clearing away the fog of unthinking and easygoing relativism, has enabled us to see evil for what it is and, more important, to celebrate the nobility of heroic courage, the dignity of civic service, and the outpouring of fellow feeling and beneficence in the wake of tragedy. It has been a long time since the mood of the country was this hospitable to serious moral reflection.

Yet the moral challenges we face in the realm of bioethics are very different from the ones confronting the nation and the world as a result of September 11. In the case of terrorism, as with slavery or despotism, it is easy to identify evil as evil; the challenge is to figure out how best to combat it. But in the realm of bioethics, the evils we face are intertwined with the goods we so keenly seek: cures for disease, relief of suffering, preservation of life. Distinguishing good and bad thus intermixed is often extremely difficult.

As champions of modern liberal democracy* we face an additional difficulty. The greatest dangers we confront in connection with the biological revolution arise not from principles alien to our way of life, but rather from those that are central to our self-definition and well-being: devotion to life and its preservation; freedom to inquire, invent or invest in whatever we want; a commitment to compassionate humanitarianism; and the confident pursuit of progress through the mastery of nature, fueled by unbridled technological advance. Yet the burgeoning technological powers to intervene in the human body and mind, justly celebrated for their contributions to human welfare, are also available for uses that could slide us down the dehumanizing path toward what C. S. Lewis called, in a power-

---

*Throughout this book, the term "liberal" is used in its classical sense, referring to regimes, societies, mores, principles and worldviews that celebrate human freedom. Its opposite is not "conservative," but "illiberal," "unfree," "totalitarian," "theocratic," or "despotic." Similarly, the term "democratic" refers to regimes, societies, mores, principles and worldviews that celebrate human equality. Its opposite is not "Republican," but "aristocratic," "hierarchic," or "monarchic." In the sense in which I use the terms, nearly all Americans, whether *ideologically* liberal or conservative, Republican or Democrat, are both "liberals" and "democrats."

ful little book by that name, the abolition of man. Thus, just as we must do battle with antimodern fanaticism and barbaric disregard for human life, so we must avoid runaway scientism and the utopian project to remake humankind in the image of our choosing. To safeguard the human future rests on our ability to steer a prudent middle course, avoiding the inhuman Osama bin Ladens on the one side and the posthuman Brave New Worlders on the other. Unfortunately, we are not yet aware of the gravity of our situation.

## Facing a Posthuman Future

The urgency of the great political struggles of the twentieth century, successfully waged against totalitarianisms of the right and of the left, seems to have blinded many people to a deeper and ultimately darker truth about the present age: nearly all contemporary societies, East as well as West, are traveling briskly in the same utopian direction. Nearly all are wedded to the modern technological project; all march eagerly to the drums of progress and fly proudly the banner of modern science; all sing loudly the Baconian anthem, "Conquer nature, relieve man's estate." Leading the triumphal procession is modern medicine, which is daily becoming ever more powerful in its battle against disease, decay and death, thanks especially to astonishing achievements in biomedical science and technology—achievements for which we must surely be grateful.

Yet contemplating present and projected advances in genetic and reproductive technologies, in neuroscience and psychopharmacology, in the development of artificial organs and computer-chip implants for human brains, and in research to retard aging, we now clearly recognize new uses for biotechnical power that soar beyond the traditional medical goals of healing disease and relieving suffering. Human nature itself lies on the operating table, ready for alteration, for eugenic and neuropsychic "enhancement," for wholesale redesign. In leading laboratories, academic and industrial, new creators are confidently amassing their powers and quietly honing their skills, while on the street their evangelists are zealously prophesying a posthuman future. For anyone who cares about preserving our humanity, the time has come to pay attention.

Some transforming powers are already here. The Pill. *In vitro* fertilization. Bottled embryos. Surrogate wombs. Cloning. Genetic screening. Genetic manipulation. Organ harvesting. Mechanical spare parts. Chimeras. Brain implants. Ritalin for the young, Viagra for the old, Prozac for everyone. And, to leave this vale of tears, a little extra morphine accompanied by Muzak.

Aldous Huxley saw it coming two generations ago. In his charming but disturbing novel *Brave New World* (it appeared in 1932 and, for me, is more powerful on each re-reading), he made its meaning strikingly visible for all to see. Unlike other frightening futuristic novels of the past century, such as Orwell's already dated *Nineteen Eighty-Four,* Huxley's portrays a dystopia that goes *with,* rather than against, the human grain. Indeed, it is animated by our most humane and progressive aspirations. Following those aspirations to their ultimate realization, Huxley enables us to recognize those less obvious but often more pernicious evils that are inextricably linked to the successful attainment of partial goods.

Huxley depicts human life seven centuries hence, living under the gentle hand of humanitarianism rendered fully competent by genetic manipulation, psychoactive drugs, hypnopaedia and high-tech amusements. At long last, mankind has succeeded in eliminating disease, aggression, war, anxiety, suffering, guilt, envy and grief. But this victory comes at the heavy price of homogenization, mediocrity, trivial pursuits, shallow attachments, debased tastes, spurious contentment and souls without loves or longings. The Brave New World has achieved prosperity, community, stability and near-universal contentment, only to be inhabited by creatures of human shape but stunted humanity. They consume, fornicate, take "soma," enjoy "centrifugal bumble-puppy," and operate the machinery that makes it all possible. They do not read, write, think, love, or govern themselves. Art and science, virtue and religion, family and friendship are all passé. What matters most is bodily health and immediate gratification: "Never put off till tomorrow the fun you can have today." No one aspires to anything higher. Brave New Man is so dehumanized that he does not even realize what has been lost.

Of course, *Brave New World* is science fiction. Our Prozac is not yet Huxley's "soma"; cloning by nuclear transfer or splitting embryos is not exactly "Bokanovskification"; MTV and virtual real-

ity parlors are not quite the "feelies"; and our current safe and con-
sequenceless sexual practices are not universally as empty or loveless as those in the novel. But the likenesses between Huxley's fictional
world and ours are disquieting, especially since our technologies of
bio-psycho-engineering are still in their infancy, yet vividly reveal
what they may look like in their full maturity. Moreover, the cultural changes that technology has already wrought among us should
make us worry even more than Huxley would have had us do.

In Huxley's novel, everything proceeds under the direction of
an omnipotent, albeit benevolent, world state. Yet the dehumanization that he depicts does not really require despotism or external
control. To the contrary, precisely because the society of the future
will deliver exactly what we most want—health, safety, comfort,
plenty, pleasure, peace of mind and length of days—we can reach
the same humanly debased condition solely by free human choice.
No need for World Controllers. Just give us the technological imperative, liberal democratic society, compassionate humanitarianism,
moral pluralism and free markets, and we can take ourselves to a
Brave New World all by ourselves—without even deliberately deciding to go. In case you haven't noticed, the train has already left the
station and is gathering speed, although there appear to be no human
hands on the throttle.

There are some who are delighted by this state of affairs: some
scientists and biotechnologists, their entrepreneurial backers and a
cheering claque of sci-fi enthusiasts, futurologists and libertarians.
There are dreams to be realized, powers to be exercised, honors to
be won and money—big money—to be made. But many of us are
worried, and not, as proponents of the revolution self-servingly
claim, because we are either ignorant of science or afraid of the
unknown. To the contrary, we can see all too clearly where the train
is headed, and we do not like the destination. We can distinguish
cleverness about means from wisdom about ends, and we are loath
to entrust the future of the race to those who cannot tell the difference. No friend of humanity cheers for a posthuman future.

Yet for all our disquiet, we have until now done nothing to
prevent it. We hide our heads in the sand because we enjoy the blessings that medicine keeps supplying, or we rationalize our inaction
by declaring that human engineering is inevitable and we cannot

stop it. In either case, we are complicit in preparing for our own degradation, and in some respects are more to blame than the bio-zealots who, however misguided, are putting their money where their mouth is. Denial and despair, unattractive outlooks in any situation, become morally reprehensible when circumstances summon us to keep the world safe for human flourishing. Our immediate ancestors, taking up the challenge of their time, rose to the occasion and rescued the human future from the cruel dehumanization of Nazi and Soviet tyranny. It is our more difficult task to find ways to preserve it from the soft dehumanization of well-meaning but hubristic biotechnical "re-creationism"—and to do it without undermining biomedical science or rejecting its genuine contributions to human welfare.

We know it will not be easy, for many features of modern life will conspire to frustrate efforts aimed toward human control of the biomedical project. First, we Americans believe in technological automatism; where we do not foolishly believe that all innovation is progress, we fatalistically believe that it is inevitable. ("If it can be done, it will be done, like it or not.") Second, we believe in freedom: the freedom of scientists to inquire, the freedom of technologists to develop, the freedom of entrepreneurs to invest and to profit, the freedom of private citizens to make use of existing technologies to satisfy any and all personal desires. Third, the biomedical enterprise occupies the moral high ground of compassionate humanitarianism, upholding the supreme values of modern life—cure disease, prolong life, relieve suffering—in competition with which other moral goods rarely stand a chance. ("What the public wants is not to be sick," says Nobel laureate James Watson, "and if we help them not to be sick, they'll be on our side.")

There are still other obstacles. Our cultural pluralism and easy-going relativism make it difficult to reach consensus on what we should embrace and what we should oppose; and serious moral objections to this or that biomedical practice are often facilely dismissed as religious or sectarian. Many people are unwilling to pronounce judgments about what is good or bad, right or wrong, even in matters of great importance, even for themselves—never mind for others or for society as a whole. It also does not help that the biomedical project is now deeply entangled with commerce: there are increasingly powerful economic interests in favor of going full steam ahead, and no economic interests in favor of going slow. Since we live in a democracy, moreover, we face political difficulties in gaining a consensus to direct our future, and we have almost no political experience in trying to curtail or even slow down the development of any new biomedical technology. Finally, and perhaps most troubling, our views of the meaning of our humanity have been so transformed by the scientific-technological approach to the world and to life that we are in danger of forgetting what we have to lose, humanly speaking.

It is this last matter to which this book is addressed. For we shall have little chance of protecting ourselves against the dangers of runaway biotechnology if we do not adequately understand what is at stake, if we do not recognize which human goods are in danger and worth defending. The first thing needful is a correction and deepening of our thinking.

## The Need for a Richer Bioethics

To be fair, judging from my students' reactions to Huxley's *Brave New World*, we are not yet so degraded or so cynical as to fail to be revolted by the society he depicts. But it is instructive to notice the nature of their objections. Sensitive egalitarians, they are bothered first by the rigid hierarchy of the cognitively stratified society, which is divided impermeably into alphas, betas, gammas, deltas and epsilons, each class with its distinctive employments and pastimes. Yet they fail to notice that, thanks to effective childhood conditioning, members of each group are utterly and equally content with their lot, so that class envy and rivalry are nonexistent. What's more, it turns out that in the end there is precious little difference between the kinds of existence enjoyed—if that is the right word— by alphas and by deltas. Everyone's needs and wants are perfectly met. Everyone is equally healthy. Regardless of class, work is utterly routine, amusements are trivial, human relations are sterile and life's most intense satisfactions come from the chemist. Indeed, one could make the case that, despite the strict distinctions of class instituted to perform the differing levels of needed technical and economic activity, the Brave New World is a more egalitarian society than our own or—let me be provocative—any other society the world has known or is likely to know. The overt inequality goes little deeper than the variously colored uniforms assigned to the different classes.

Because we are liberals as well as egalitarians, our second complaint is about a lack of freedom. Everyone's endowments are predetermined through genetic engineering, all beliefs are conditioned, and conformity is obligatory. Using high-powered psychological and chemical techniques of behavior management, the World Controllers see to it that nothing disturbs the peace or social stability, and all deviants and misfits who think for themselves are whisked away to an island to live among their kind. Huxley himself apparently regarded the absence of freedom as the central problem of his dystopia: the epigraph he selected for the novel is a passage from Nicholas Berdiaeff predicting that the world's elite will soon turn its back on the march to utopia, calling instead for a society "less 'perfect,' and more free."

Yet the lack of freedom, while serious, is *not* the central defect. People with freedom are capable, entirely of their own volition, of embracing the same shallow relationships and trivial pursuits as the denizens of Brave New World. If you require proof, just look around. To be sure, while freedom is a great desideratum, it is no firewall against willful self-debasement. Everything will depend, finally, not just on the possibility of choice, but on what is chosen. What is most repulsive about the Brave New World is not inequality or lack of freedom, but dehumanization and degradation—and, worst of all, that their posthuman estate is neither regretted nor recognized by anyone, and that they aspire to nothing humanly richer or higher. To the extent that we readers also cannot discern the dehumanization in Huxley's portrait, we are already more than halfway to it.

Our blindness to the signs and symptoms of dehumanization is, unfortunately, not confined to our work as literary critics of Huxley's novel. It also keeps us from noticing the deepest dangers connected with the brave new biology. Most troubling, this blindness is endemic even among American bioethicists, those whose profession it is to teach us about the meaning of the biotechnologies now being perfected, week by week, day by day. So little disquieted are mainstream bioethicists by what is coming that they have entered in large numbers into the employ of the biotechnology companies, bestowing their moral blessings on the latest innovation—assuredly not for love but for money. If these "experts" can't see or don't care about what lies ahead, what hope is there for the rest of us?

The major principles of professional bioethics, according to the profession's own self-declaration, are these: (1) beneficence (or at least "nonmaleficence"—in plain English, "do no harm"), (2) respect for persons, and (3) justice. As applied to particular cases, these principles translate mainly into concerns to avoid bodily harm and do bodily good, to respect patient autonomy and secure informed consent, and to promote equal access to health care and provide equal protection against biohazards. So long as nobody is hurt, no one's will is violated, and no one is excluded or discriminated against, there is little to worry about. The possibility of willing dehumanization is out of sight and out of mind.

Consider some of our recent bioethical debates: First, embryonic stem cell research, where the question was argued almost entirely in terms of the goods of life and health. Those in favor insisted that regenerative medicine using stem cells will eventually save countless lives and eliminate crushing incapacity; those opposed insisted that, in the meantime, lives would be sacrificed in the process, the lives of human embryos now stored in the freezers of *in vitro* fertilization clinics. Few people paid attention to the meaning of using the seeds of the next generation as a tool for saving the lives of the present one. (Consider as a parable in this regard the hypothetical case of the last couple on earth, he with Alzheimer's disease, she with exactly two embryos that could be used either to produce stem cells for the husband or to start the renewal of the human race.) Fewer people yet worried about the effects not on the embryos but on our embryo-using society of coming to look upon nascent human life as a natural resource to be mined, exploited, commodified. The little embryos are merely destroyed, but we—their users—are at risk of corruption. We are desensitized and denatured by a coarsening of sensibility that comes to regard these practices as natural, ordinary and fully unproblematic. People who can hold nascent human life in their hands coolly and without awe have deadened something in their souls.

Or take human cloning. President Clinton's National Bioethics Advisory Commission, in its 1997 report *Cloning Human Beings,* could agree only that human cloning is for now unethical, because it is, for now, unsafe—an important objection, to be sure, but, note well, not an objection to *cloning itself*. Against these advisors stand the libertarians, who insist that all judgments about cloning or other novel forms of baby-making should be viewed solely as matters of private reproductive choice: in a free country, people have a right to reproduce by whatever means they wish, and regardless of who thinks otherwise. By and large, both these groups have pooh-poohed as irrational the widespread public repugnance to this prospect, choosing to prefer their reasonings and rationalizations to what might be a deeper, if inarticulate, wisdom. The bioethicists, whether libertarian, egalitarian or humanitarian, are by and large unconcerned with the positive good of keeping human procreation human, of upholding the difference between procreation and manufacture, between begetting and making. Few of them ponder what it will mean for the relation between the generations when children do not arise from the coupling of two but from the replication of one. Few seem to care about what it means for a society increasingly to regard a child not as a mysterious stranger given to be cherished as someone to take our place, but rather as a product of our will, to be perfected by design and to satisfy our wants.

Or take allowing commerce in organs for transplantation, a prospect now making a comeback in the United States after almost two decades of legal proscription. Once again, the battle is between the patrons of life and the patrons of justice: on the one hand, financial incentives will increase the supply of organs, hence fewer will die; on the other hand, financial incentives will lead to the exploitation of the desperately poor, compounding the injustice of their already unjust condition. Few people seem to be concerned about the implications of regarding the human body as alienable property or what all this bodes for ideas of human wholeness, identity and personal dignity.

Or take the coming knowledge of the human genome and the prospect of universal genetic screening and genetic engineering, including so-called germ-line modifications that will directly and deliberately affect future generations. In the United States the dominant ethical discussions are about genetic discrimination in insurance or employment and the matter of "genetic privacy." No one talks much about the hazards to living humanly from knowing *too much* about your genetic future. No one talks much about the meaning of acquiring godlike powers of deciding which genetic sins are capital offenses against the holy ghost of Health. No one talks much about the dangers of eugenics. No one talks at all about the hubris of believing that we are now, or ever can be, wise enough to use these powers to engineer "improvements" in the next generation.

Finally, take the use of drugs to enhance performance—in sports, at school, or in the current crude replacement for what used to be called courtship. There are concerns about taking unfair advantage of an athletic rival (steroids and "blood doping") or an attractive female ("Ecstasy"), and there are concerns about coercive pacification of children by authorities (the misuse of Ritalin in schools). But there is little attention to what it means to begin to change the deep structure of human activity, severing performance from effort or, in other cases, pleasure from the activity that ordinarily is its foundation. We worry about addiction to powerful drugs and the bodily harm it causes or the crimes that are related to the fact that they are illegal. But we have yet to recognize the transformation in our humanity that would come from disturbing, through drugs or brain implants, our fundamental ways of encountering, enjoying, and acting in and on the world.

In a word, we are quick to notice dangers to life, threats to freedom, risks of discrimination or exploitation of the poor, and interference with anyone's pursuit of pleasure. But we are slow to recognize threats to human dignity, to the ways of doing and feeling and being in the world that make human life rich, deep and fulfilling.

## The Strengths and Limits of Liberal Principles

That this is so ought to be no surprise, given who we are. We come by this outlook honestly, for we are liberals and we are democrats (both lowercase). We are the privileged descendants of wise Founders who, in declaring independence from the mother country, defined themselves (and us) as a people by holding as self-evidently true that all men are created equal, equally endowed with the inalienable rights of life, liberty and the pursuit of happiness; and, further, that governments exist among men (solely) to secure these rights against the depredations of princes, prelates and their minions, or anyone else who might seek to deny them.

It is impossible to exaggerate the debt we Americans and the world at large owe to the political triumph of these liberal democratic principles. Thanks to liberal democracy and its fruitful contract with modern science and technology, many ordinary human beings today live healthier, longer, freer, safer and more prosperous lives than did most dukes and princes in premodern times. And yet—though it may appear ungrateful to do so, especially when modern liberal societies have so recently come under lethal attack from religious zealots—we must acknowledge that these liberal principles by themselves are inadequate for dealing with the threats of the brave new biology. For one thing, as we shall soon see, they neglect other worthy goods without which human life will not remain human. For another, they easily become a debased coinage and contribute to the forces that make a brave new world seem attractive and render its arrival more likely.

The liberal principles were, to begin with, narrowly political. The rights of the Declaration of Independence were asserted to protect against despotism, not to serve as sole moral tender in all social matters and private life. Here, morals and mores were rather to be informed by biblical religion, the source of a richer and fuller teaching about the whole of human life. Though the national government eschewed religious establishment or religious tests for office, the Founders were not neutral as between religion and irreligion, and several of the individual states had established churches. Yet as the nation has become more pluralistic and more secularized, and as the once merely political language of rights has invaded and come to dominate all moral discourse, the liberal principles have been transformed—and, in my view, corrupted—by expansion and exaggeration. Here's how:

Beyond an obligation to protect life against foreign enemies and local murderers, we now believe government has an obligation to preserve life from disease and to provide requisite health care. The fear of violent death, a root passion of liberalism that inspired men to abolish feudal and religious politics with their penchant for endless civil war, has become the fear of death altogether, summoning science and medicine to do battle with mortality itself as if death were but one more disease—through hormones, regenerative medicine using stem cells, and attempts to reset the genetic clock that sets the midnight hour on the maximum human lifespan. From liberty understood first as freedom of conscience and the negative right not to suffer under the rule of despots has come liberty understood as a positive right to self-expression, self-assertion and full self-re-creation. In a moral realm impoverished by an overgrowth of rights, liberty is indistinguishable from license and becomes perfectly compatible with licentiousness. The liberty of self-assertion is even said to include the right of assisted suicide, the self-contradictory freedom to choose no longer to be a choosing creature. The inalienable right to own property has now become a right to alienate parts of one's own body *as* property. Living human embryos, if produced with the aid of genetic manipulation, are now patentable matter, and we are but a small step from instituting the buying and selling of body parts. Property, a right grounded in the inalienable "my-own-ness" of my body and its labor, has given rise to ideas of commodifying the body itself. Older pre- or nonliberal notions of human dignity, formerly the social counterweight to the political doctrine of rights, have been greatly attenuated—partly thanks to the success of liberalism and its alliance with the modern technological project for the mastery of nature. The right to the pursuit of happiness—that is, to the *practice* of happiness, to living one's life as one sees fit—is, as a result, perfectly compatible with utter self-indulgence, mindless pastimes and the factitious gratifications of high-tech amusements and drug-induced euphoria. Anyone for Brave New World? Why not.

What is missing from the liberal pantheon of goods, especially in their postmodern version? What goods besides life, liberty and the pursuit of happiness do we seek to defend? What has been lost when we find degradation, debasement and dehumanization? As I have already indicated several times, the obvious candidate is "human dignity"—a term we sometimes pair with "human freedom," implying (we are dimly aware) that human freedom is not the only good worth defending. Human dignity is in fact a useful notion, perhaps even the right one, and I confess to making much use of it myself. Yet if it is to be more than an empty slogan, we need to articulate its meaning, and in ways accessible and persuasive to our fellow citizens. This is no easy matter.

## *The Search for Human Dignity*

The first trouble with "dignity" is that it is an abstraction, and a soft one at that. "Harm" is another abstraction, but we do not lack for concrete examples: a broken bone, a burned-down house, a stolen purse. "Dignity" is much more elusive, so much so that many in the field of bioethics mock it or treat it as a merely "symbolic" value—meaning that it has no concrete reality. With some effort, these difficulties can be negotiated; but then the real trouble starts, because not everyone agrees about the nature and ground of human dignity.

Dignity is, to begin with, an undemocratic idea. The central notion etymologically, both in English and in its Latin root (*dignitas*), is that of worthiness, elevation, honor, nobility, height—in short, of excellence or virtue. In all its meanings it is a term of distinction; dignity is not something that, like a nose or a navel, is to be expected or found in every living human being. Dignity would seem to be, in principle, aristocratic.

Though they did not have the term, dignity as honor linked to excellence or virtue would certainly be the view of the ancient Greeks. In the heroic world of the poets, the true or full human being, the he-man who drew honor and prizes as his dignity, displayed his worthiness in noble and glorious deeds. Supreme was the virtue of courage: the willingness to face death in battle, armed only with your own prowess, going forth against an equally worthy opponent who, like you, sought a victory not only over the adversary but, as it were, over death itself. This heroic dignity—think Achilles and Hector—is poles apart from the bourgeois fear of death and love of medicine, though, paradoxically, it honored the human body as a thing of beauty to a degree unsurpassed in human history. Later, following the Socratic turn, heroic excellence was supplanted in Greek philosophy by the virtue of wisdom; the new hero was not the glorious warrior but the man singularly devoted to wisdom, living close to death not on the field of battle but by a single-minded quest for knowledge eternal.

The heroic warrior and the courageous wisdom-seeker may indeed be pinnacles of human dignity; we today still read about Achilles and Socrates with admiration. But the Greek exemplars are of little practical use in democratic times. Moreover, the problem with Brave New World is not primarily that it lacks glorious warriors or outstanding philosophers (or artists or scientists or statesmen)—although the fact that they are not appreciated in such a world is telling. The basic problem is the absence of a kind of human dignity more abundantly found and universally shared.

In the Western philosophical tradition, the most high-minded attempt to supply a teaching of universal human dignity belongs to Kant, with his doctrine of respect for *persons*. Persons—*all* persons or rational beings—are deserving of respect not because of some realized excellence of achievement, but because of a universally shared participation in morality and the ability to live under the moral law. However we may finally judge it, there is something highly dignified in Kant's project. For he strained every nerve to find and preserve a place for human freedom and dignity in the face of the Newtonian worldview, a mechanized account of nature that captured even the human being, omitting only his rational will. And, in its content, there is something austerely dignified in the Kantian refusal to confuse reason with rationalization, duty with inclination, and the right and the good with happiness (pleasure). Whatever persists of a nonutilitarian ethic in contemporary bioethics descends from this principled, moralistic view. The respect for persons so widely celebrated in the canons of ethics governing human experimentation is in fact a descendant of Kant's principle of human autonomy. Never mind that for most people, human autonomy no longer means living under the universalizable law that self-legislating reason prescribes for itself, but has come to mean "choosing for yourself, whatever you choose," or even "asserting yourself authentically, reason be damned." Lurking even in this debased view of the "autonomous person" is an idea of man as something more than a bundle of impulses seeking release and a bag of itches seeking scratching. "Personhood," understood as genuine moral agency, is indeed threatened by powers to engineer our genetic makeup and to fiddle around with human appetites through psychoactive drugs or implanting computer chips in brains. We are not wrong to seek to protect it.

Yet this view of human dignity is finally very inadequate, not because it is undemocratic but because it is, in an important respect, *inhuman*. Precisely because it dualistically sets up the concept of "personhood" *in opposition* to nature and the body, it fails to do justice to the concrete reality of our embodied lives—lives of begetting and belonging no less than of willing and thinking. Precisely because it is universalistically rational, it denies the importance of life's concrete particularity, lived always locally, corporeally, and in a unique trajectory from zygote in the womb to body in the coffin. Precisely because "personhood" is distinct from our lives as embodied, rooted, connected and aspiring beings, the dignity of rational choice pays no respect at all to the dignity we have through our loves and longings—central aspects of human life understood as a grown togetherness of body and soul. Not all of human dignity consists in reason or freedom.

It is easy to see why the notion of "personal dignity" is of limited value in the realm of bioethics. As one would predict, the bioethics of personhood is very good at defending those aspects of human dignity tied to respect for autonomy against violations of human will, including failures to gain informed consent and excessively paternalistic behavior by experts and physicians. The justly celebrated canons of ethics governing human experimentation are, in fact, descendants of Kant's principle of human autonomy and the need to protect the weak against the powerful. But this moral teaching has very little to offer us in the battle against the dehumanizing hazards of a Brave New World. For it is, in fact, perfectly comfortable with embryo farming, surrogate motherhood, cloning, the sale of organs, or even extracorporeal gestation, because these peculiar treatments of the body or uses of our embodiments are no harm to that homunculus of personhood that resides somewhere happily in a morally disembodied place. *Pace* Kant, the answer for the threat to human dignity arising from sacrificing the high to the urgent, the soul to the body, is not a teaching of human dignity that severs mind from body, that ignores the urgent, or that denies dignity to human bodily life as lived. The defense of what is humanly high requires an equal defense of what is seemingly low.

The account of *human* dignity we seek goes beyond the said dignity of "persons," to reflect and embrace the worthiness of embodied human life, and therewith of our natural desires and passions, our natural origins and attachments, our sentiments and aversions, our loves and longings. What we need is a defense of the dignity of what Tolstoy called "real life," life as ordinarily lived, everyday life in its concreteness. It is a life lived always with and against necessity, struggling to meet it, not to eliminate it. Like the downward pull of gravity without which the dancer cannot dance, the downward pull of bodily necessity and fate makes possible the dignified journey of a truly human life. It is a life that will use our awareness of need, limitation and mortality to craft a way of being that has engagement, depth, beauty, virtue and meaning—not despite our embodiment but *because* of it. Human aspiration depends absolutely on our being creatures of need and finitude, and hence of longings and attachments.

Sophisticated modern liberals will have a hard time with such a suggestion. What, they may well ask, is so dignified about our embodiment? What is inherently dignified about human procreation? What is so dignified in the fact that we rise from the union of egg and sperm, grow as an embryo and fetus in the darkness of a womb, or enter the world through the birth canal—all rather messy matters, truth to tell—rather than, say, as a result of being designed perfectly in the light of a tidy laboratory? What is so dignified about being the product of chance rather than rational design? Of natural sex rather than human artfulness? What would be wrong with cloning or any other sexless form of making babies?

Or, turning from procreation to the rest of life, what is so dignified about having a body that is subject to disease and decay? Given its inherent limitations, what's wrong with regarding it instrumentally as a tool, rather than pretending that it is a temple? What could be wrong with replacing its worn-out parts, as one does with an aging machine? And why should we not do everything in our power to combat the body's corruption, including especially its ultimate mortal fate? What is so dignified about the fact that, thanks to this mortal coil of flesh, we must die leaving no earthly trace?

Finding good answers to these tough questions is the deepest challenge for a truly human bioethics, one that seeks to keep human life human. Answers depend not on science or even on ethics but on a proper anthropology, one that richly understands what it means to be a human animal, in our bodily, psychic, social, cultural, political, and spiritual dimensions. For we cannot even begin to discuss the possible dignity of human embodiment, human procreation or human finitude if we do not seek to grasp their being and meaning. While I do not even pretend to tackle the job head on, I will broach these anthropological issues in the chapters to come, and will offer some insights and suggestions that may point the way to the right sort of account. For the time being, however, let the following remarks serve as an invitation.

It was not an accident that Aldous Huxley introduced us to the Brave New World by inviting us into the fertilizing room of the Central London Hatchery, where new human life is produced to order outside the body and cloning is routine. It was not an accident that "birth" and "mother" are regarded in that society as smutty notions. For there is a deep connection between these perversions of our bodily beginnings and attachments and the degraded flatness of soul that characterizes the entire society Huxley depicts. Why? Because to say "yes" to baby manufacture is to say "no" to all natural human relations, is to say "no" also to the deepest meaning of human sexual coupling, namely, human *erotic* longing. For human *eros* is the fruit of the peculiar conjunction of and competition between two divergent aspirations within a single living body, the impulse to self-preservation and the urge to reproduce. The first is a self-regarding concern for our own personal permanence and satisfaction; the second is a self-denying aspiration for something that transcends our own finite existence, and for the sake of which we spend and even give our lives. Other animals, of course, live with these twin and opposing drives. But only the human animal is conscious of their existence and is driven to devise a life based in part on the tension between them, in part on the fact that he does not fully understand what it is that his embodied life "wants of him." In consequence, only the human animal has explicit and conscious longings for something higher, something whole, something eternal, longings that we would not have were we not the conjunction of this bodily "doubleness," elevated and directed upwards through conscious self-awareness. Nothing humanly fine, let alone great, will come out of a society that has crushed the source of human aspiration, the germ of which is to be found in the meaning of the sexually complementary "two" that seek unity and wholeness, and willingly devote themselves to the well-being of their offspring. Nothing humanly fine, let alone great, will come out of a society that is willing to sacrifice all other goods to keep the present generation alive and intact. Nothing humanly fine, let alone great, will come from the desire to pursue bodily immortality for ourselves.

Finding our way to such insights is, I admit, an increasingly difficult task in modern America. A culture that offers endless remedies to prolong the lives of the living is less likely to be a culture devoted to or interested in procreation. A society, when it does procreate, that sees its children as projects rather than as gifts is unlikely even to be open to the question of the meaning and dignity of procreation. And a culture instructed about life by a biology that sees whole organisms mainly in terms of parts or, what's worse, as mere instruments for the perpetuation of genes—"a chicken is just a gene's way of making more genes"—will reject the question of meaning altogether, because it believes that it already has the answer.

Here at last we have come to the bottom of our troubles. It turns out that the most fundamental challenge posed by the brave new biology comes not from the biotechnologies it spawns, but from the underlying scientific thought. In order effectively to serve the needs of human life, modern biology reconceived the nature of the organic body, representing it not as something animated, purposive and striving, but as dead matter-in-motion. This reductive science has given us enormous power, but it offers us no standards to guide its use. Worse, it challenges our self-understanding as creatures of dignity, rendering us incapable of recognizing dangers to our humanity that arise from the very triumphs biology has made. What is urgently needed is a richer, more natural biology and anthropology, one that does full justice to the meaning of our peculiarly human union of soul and body in which low neediness and divine-seeking aspiration are concretely joined.

In our search for such an account, we can get help from premodern sources, both philosophical and biblical. We can learn, for example, from Aristotle an account of soul that is not a ghost in the machine, but the empowered form of a naturally organic body. We can learn from thinking about Genesis what it means that the earth's most godlike creature is a concretion combining ruddy earth and rosying breath; why it is not good for the man to be alone; why the remedy for man's aloneness is a sexual counterpart, not a dialectic partner (Eve, not Socrates); why in the shame-filled discovery of sexual nakedness is humanity's first awe-filled awareness of the divine; and why respect for a being created in God's image means respecting *everything* about him, not just his freedom or his reason but also his blood. Exploring these possibilities is for another volume. For now it will be sufficient if we can come to see the need for both a new bioethics and a new biology: a richer ethic of *bios* tied to a richer *logos* of *bios,* an ethical account of human flourishing based on a biological account of human life as lived, not just physically, but psychically, socially and spiritually. In the absence of such an account we shall not be able to meet the dehumanizing challenges of the brave new biology.

Despite the dark picture I have sketched, things are not so dark on the ground. It may be that human dignity has a future, needing only some encouragement and voice for what many people still know in their bones. The events of September 11 have reminded us that courage, fortitude, generosity, righteousness and the other human virtues are not confined solely to the few. Many of us strive for them, with partial success, and still more of us do ourselves honor when we recognize and admire those people nobler and finer than ourselves. With proper models, proper rearing and proper encouragement, many of us can be and act more in accord with our higher natures.

In truth, if we know how to look, we find evidence of human dignity all around us, in the valiant efforts ordinary people make to meet necessity, to combat adversity and disappointment, to provide for their children, to care for their parents, to help their neighbors, to serve their country. Life provides numerous hard occasions that call for endurance and equanimity, generosity and kindness, courage and self-command. Adversity sometimes brings out the best in a man, and often shows best what he is made of. Confronting our own death—or the deaths of our beloved ones—provides an opportunity for the exercise of our humanity, for the great and small alike. Profoundly should we hope and pray that the recent shocking reminder of the vulnerability of all things human, and the recent stirring display of the dignity of ordinary human heroes, will encourage us to come to dignity's defense also against the seductive temptations of a posthuman future.

## An Overview of the Argument

It remains here only for me to introduce the structure of the book, to offer a synopsis of its argument, and to say a word about its spirit. The surface thesis has already been stated: the new biotechnologies threaten not so much liberty and equality as something we might summarily call "human dignity." Technology has done, and will likely continue to do, wonders for our health and longevity, for the defense of our freedom and for our prosperity ("Life, Liberty and the Pursuit of Happiness"). Yet it threatens human flourishing precisely because, in the absence of countervailing efforts, we may use the fear of death, our various freedoms and rights, and our unrestrained pursuit of profit and pleasure in ways that will make us into human midgets. Our embrace of technology would thus turn out to be tragic, unless we redeem ourselves by nontechnological ideas and practices, today both increasingly beleaguered.

The first section of the book, *Nature and Purposes of Technology and Ethics,* examines in general terms the two poles of our discussion: technology and ethics. Chapter One lays out "The Problem of Technology and Liberal Democracy" in a comprehensive statement, showing what I mean by suggesting that technology is not so much "problem" as "tragedy." Chapter Two, "Practicing Ethics: Where's the Action?" dissects the current fashions in ethics and bioethics, and shows why they are woefully inadequate to the task of a truly human response to our new predicament, both in action and in thought.

The second and longest section of the book, *Ethical Challenges from Biotechnology,* moves through selected areas of biomedical science and technology, from *in vitro* fertilization and genetic technology to organ transplantation and "immortality research." Its purpose is to expose the challenges that these new developments pose to life and lineage, identity and individuality, bodily unity and integrity, the dignity of the body, the care of the dying, and the virtues that we possess only thanks to our mortal condition. Within this section are three subsections: *Life and Lineage: Genetics and the Beginning of Life* (Chapters Three to Five); *Body and Soul: Parts and Whole in the Midst of Life* (Chapter Six); and *Death and Immortality: Staying Human at the End of Life* (Chapters Seven to Nine).

Chapter Three, "The Meaning of Life—in the Laboratory," starts with the germinal beginnings of life and our abilities to manipulate them, both for producing children and for biomedical research. It focuses on the meaning of holding embryonic life in human hands and the temptation to reduce it to raw material for human use, exploitation and commerce.

Chapter Four, "The Age of Genetic Technology Arrives," looks at some of the implications of the human genome project and the coming prospects for genetic screening and genetic engineering, serving purposes both therapeutic and beyond. It defends the reasonableness of public disquiet regarding the dangers of "playing God," of coercion and especially of dehumanization—in both deed and thought—that are raised by prospects of genetic "enhancement" and by an approach to human life that defines us in terms of our genes.

Chapter Five, "Cloning and the Posthuman Future," examines the much-discussed matter of human cloning. It treats this as the opening gambit of a eugenic campaign of thought and action, one that would turn procreation into manufacture and have us treat children (even more than we already do) as planned products to be perfected rather than as mysterious gifts to be treasured. Recommendation of a legislative ban on all human cloning self-consciously argues in the name of human dignity for the need to set limits on human freedom, both regarding what scientists may do and regarding how babies are to be "made."

Chapter Six, "Organs for Sale? Propriety, Property and the Price of Progress," looks at proposals to establish markets in organs for transplantation. It exposes the implications for our sense of identity and integrity of our death-defying commercial republic's growing willingness to turn all human body parts into commodities, replacing an ethos of love and philanthropic gifting of organs with an ethos of rent-seeking behavior—in human flesh. The right of property and the freedom of contract, central liberal notions, are shown to be insufficient protectors of human dignity.

Chapter Seven, "Is There a Right to Die?" continues the critique of liberal rights, this time not the right to property in organs in the name of saving life, but the alleged new right to be made dead (with the deadly assistance of others), if one wants out of life. Here the perversions of a rights-based approach to all moral questions are made clear for all to see, threatening even the dignity and well-being of the dying patients that the alleged "right to die" is intended to benefit.

Chapter Eight, "Death with Dignity and the Sanctity of Life," the only chapter that thematically treats the idea of "dignity," provides a better alternative than "right to die" approaches to thinking about how to care for people at the end of life. The major focus here is to show how the dignity of life and the sanctity of life are conjoined, preparing the ground for the fusion of the perspectives of virtue and the perspectives of reverence.

Chapter Nine, "*L'Chaim* and Its Limits: Why Not Immortality?" grabs the biotechnology bull by the horns, countering proposals that we pursue the conquest of death itself with arguments against our insatiable lust for unending life. Central to the case is an attempt to articulate what a dignified human life is all about: engagement, seriousness, the love of beauty, the practice of moral virtue, the aspiration to something transcendent, the love of understanding, the gift of children and the possibility of perpetuating a life devoted to a high and holy calling.

The third section of the book, *Nature and Purposes of Biology,* draws back from the biotechnologies to have a brief look at the underlying scientific quest. Chapter Ten, "The Permanent Limitations of Biology," develops the thought that the deepest threat to human dignity lies not in the techniques of biotechnology but in the underlying science itself, in an "objectified" treatment of life that fails to do justice to its subject. The chapter's purpose is to induce humility where there is now only epistemological hubris, and to recreate a sense of wonder and mystery about the world, a reverential contemplative attitude that is itself an expression of human dignity. For man is the only being on earth that can experience wonder and awe at the rich and incredible facts of life, soul and human awareness. A restoration of appreciative wonder and respectful awe before the mystery of life is indispensable if we are to be able to defend life's dignity against the deadly distortions of scientistic abstraction.

Finally, a word of warning about the spirit of this book. I fear that nothing I can say will prevent many readers of this book from regarding it as a Luddite tract, and me as hostile to science and technology, or a natural pessimist, or someone simply fearful of the future. Only to the last do I plead guilty—and then only in part—though not as a matter of temperament or psychic flaw, but because the evidence seems to me to require deep moral concern about the direction we are pursuing. As to the other charges, I simply flat-out deny them.

I regard modern science as one of the great monuments to the human intellect, and the field of modern biology as unrivalled in the wonderful discoveries it can and will increasingly offer us. I esteem greatly modern medicine for its contributions to human well-being, even where—for example, with organ transplantation or *in vitro* fertilization—I am willing to call attention to some moral hazards. And I am profoundly grateful, both personally and philanthropically, to modern American democracy for its safeguarding of life and liberty, equal opportunity and prosperity, and, above all, for the unprecedented opportunities of modern life to educate ourselves and to make something humanly fine and good out of our precious lives. If people wish to accuse me of being antiscience, I respectfully submit that the problem is theirs.

Scientists and physicians, unused to thinking that their work is anything but self-justifying, may balk at suggestions that their work may not be unqualifiedly good in its results. Confirmed materialists will see the threat of theocracy hiding behind any challenge to the sufficiency of their explanations of the world. Doctrinaire libertarians will not consider that freedom can lead us anywhere but upward. Prosperous sophisticates cannot imagine that they are missing anything important in the beliefs to which they are so comfortably attached: "We are living well; what reason is there to worry?" But that is precisely the problem. The heart of the *possibility* of tragedy is that human glory and human misery are linked, that the triumph of human achievement contains intrinsically the source of human degradation. And the *likelihood* of *suffering* tragedy increases with a hubristic belief that we have everything under control. If I have written too polemically, it is only because of a passionate concern that we consider before it is too late whether we truly know what we are doing. Anyone who cares for the future of human dignity no less than for the future of human health should not want to be self-deceived in this matter. It is to encourage greater thoughtfulness in such readers that I have written this book.

# ❋ Nature and Purposes of Technology and Ethics

# CHAPTER ONE

# The Problem of Technology and Liberal Democracy

"Biotechnology" is a neologism for the new age. New and novel also is the thing it names: industrial-scale processes and products offering power to alter and control the phenomena of life—in plants, in animals and, increasingly, also in human beings. But while the word may be new, the *idea* of biotechnology is old, and so are the motives behind it. It is central to the modern humanistic vision, first conjured in the seventeenth century, that would bring the pursuit of knowledge into firm marriage with the aspirations of humankind for the conquest of disease, the relief of suffering and the prolongation of life.

As I have already said, biotechnology today flourishes especially in liberal democracies. Its practice takes advantage of their freedoms; its products serve the needs of multitudes. Yet as I will argue from start to finish in this book, biotechnology and the science on which it rests are proving to be a growing problem for liberal democracies, both in practice and in thought. To understand why this might be so, it is helpful to place biotechnology in its larger context and to consider more generally the problem of technology as a whole.

Attempting an overview of the problem of technology is daunting. For one thing, the topic is enormous: technology is everywhere, in a shifting variety of guises, from flush toilets to food processors, from automobiles to artificial organs, from cell phones to smart bombs. Second, given this vast heterogeneity, it seems foolish to try to identify *the* problem of technology, let alone how it relates to liberal democracy, a hefty subject by itself. Third, there is the embarrassment of apparent hypocrisy: how can a man who travels hither and yon by airplane and automobile, to deliver lectures produced on a computer and laser printer, rendered legible and audible through eyeglasses and microphone, and now made readable through the latest printing and publishing techniques, have the effrontery to speak about technology as a problem? Finally, there is the matter of my limited competence; though I have worried for more than thirty years about the meaning of biomedical technologies, I remain largely ignorant of other technological areas and, I confess, I have not often tried to think about the problem of technology whole.

Still, one must make the attempt, for the stakes are high. For one suspects that technology, despite its great diversity, remains in some sense "a whole," whose aggregate significance for human life cannot be exaggerated. We have lost our innocence about technology in recent decades, and hence we need all the more to try to understand it.

Probably the most common view of "the problem of technology" is something like this: technology is the sum total of human tools and methods, devised by human beings to control our environment for our own benefit. Because it is essentially *instrumental,* technology is itself morally neutral, usable for both good and ill. There are, of course, dangers of abuse and misuse of technology, but these appear to be problems not of technology but of its human users, to be addressed by morality in general. And, besides abuse and misuse, there is a genuine problem of technology itself: the unintended and undesired consequences arising from its *proper* use. Thus, the problems of technology can be dealt with, on one side, by technology assessment and careful regulation (to handle side effects and misuse), and, on the other side, by good will, compassion, and the love of humanity (to prevent abuse). This combination will enable us to solve the problems technology creates without sacrificing its delightful fruits.

This view, I contend, is much too simple. It holds too narrow an understanding of the nature of technology, too shallow a view of the difficulties it produces, and too optimistic a view of our ability to deal with them—not least because this vision is itself infected with the problem of technology. That at least is what I will now endeavor to show.

## What Is Technology?

We must begin by trying to understand what technology is. The term itself is singularly unhelpful; according to the *Oxford English Dictionary*, its original English meaning, dating back to the early seventeenth century, was "a discourse or treatise [that is, a *logos*] on art or the arts," or, again, "the scientific study [a *logos*] of the practical or industrial arts." A second meaning identifies technology as "technical nomenclature," that is, the terminology or speech—*logos*—of a particular art. Only in the nineteenth century was the meaning transferred to the practical arts themselves, taken collectively: "His technology consists of weaving, cutting canoes, making rude weapons" (1864).

The term has Greek roots: *techne,* meaning art, especially the useful crafts rather than the fine arts, that is, carpentry and shoemaking rather than poetry and dance; and *logos,* meaning articulate speech or discursive reason. But the Greeks did not have the compound *technologos.* As far as I can tell, the closest they came to any such notion was not an account about art—a *logos* of *techne*—but an art of speaking. Rhetoric, the art of persuasive speech, was indeed a *techne* of *logos,* and in the Sophists' view a means of rationalizing political life free of the need for force.[1] (One could, I think, get very far in understanding the difference between the ancient Greek polis and the modern nation-state by beginning with and thinking through the difference between technology understood as *rhetoric* and technology understood as *rationalized art and industry.*)

Still, art and speech are intimately related. Both are manifestations of human rationality, of the fact that man is the animal having *logos,* the rational or reasoning animal. Human craft, unlike the productive activities of animals, is not spontaneous or instinctive. It involves deliberating, calculating, ordering, thinking, planning—all manifestations of *logos.* The connection was observed succinctly by Aristotle: *techne,* he said, is a disposition or habit of *making* (as contrasted with doing) involving true reasoning (*logos*).[2] All artful making has a manual element, to be sure, but to be truly technical it must be guided by mind, know-how, expertise. It is this mental and rational element that makes the various arts eminently teachable—through various "how-to" guides and manuals. (About the *disposition* to make—that is, why human beings *want* to make—I will speak shortly.) Following up these clues, one might think that technology is the sum of the products of craft and industry, and, even more, the sum of the know-how, skills and other devices for their production and use.

But this is, at best, a partial view. Technology, especially modern technology, occupies itself not only with the bringing-into-being of machines and tools and other artifacts. It is centrally involved in the harnessing of power and energy—thermal, hydroelectric, chemical, solar, atomic. The drilling for oil, the damming of rivers, the splitting of atoms provide not objects of art but an undifferentiated ready resource for all sorts of human activities, both in war and in peace. Indeed, according to Heidegger, this aspect of modern technology is essential and decisive. Modern technology is less a bringing forth of objects than a setting upon, a challenging forth, a demanding of nature: that its concealed materials and energies be released and ordered as standing reserves, available and transformable for any multitude of purposes.[3] Not the loom or the plow, but the oil storage tank or the steel mill or the dynamo, is the emblem of modern technology.

Yet this, too, does not go far enough. For technology and technique are not today limited to external and physical nature; technology now works directly on the technologist, on man himself. There is burgeoning biomedical technology, to this point largely harnessed by the art of healing, but in the future usable also for genetic engineering and the like. There is psychological technology, from various techniques of psychotherapy to psychopharmacology. There are abundant techniques of education, communication and entertainment; techniques of social organization and engineering (for example, the army and the police); techniques of management (the factory or the boardroom); techniques of inspection and regulation; techniques of selling and buying, learning and rearing, dating and mating, birthing and dying, and even—God help us—of grief. In modern times, as Jacques Ellul has persuasively argued, the technical is ubiquitous, much wider and deeper than the mechanical or the energetic. For him (as for Heidegger), technology is an entire way of being in the world, a social phenomenon more than a merely material one, characterized by the effort, through rational analysis, methodical artfulness and correlative organization, to order all aspects of our world toward efficiency, ease and control—to achieve the fullest control at the highest efficiency at the least possible cost and trouble.[4] Technology comprises organization and scheduling no less than machinery and fuel, concepts and methods no less than physical processes. In short, it is a way of thinking and believing and feeling, a way of standing in and toward the world. Technology, in its full meaning, is the disposition rationally to order and predict and control everything feasible in order to master fortune and spontaneity, violence and wildness, and leave nothing to chance, all for human benefit. It is technology thus understood, as the disposition to rational mastery, whose problem we hope to discover.

Whence comes such a disposition to mastery? What is the source of the technological attitude? Again, a question difficult to unravel. According to some, its deepest roots are somehow tied to human weakness: necessity is the mother of invention. Need lies behind the fishhook and the plow, fear of beasts and men behind the club and the barricade, and fear of death behind medicine. It is, according to Hobbes, the fear of violent death that awakens human reason and the quest for mastery. Of course, too much fear can enervate. According to Aeschylus's Prometheus, only when men ceased seeing doom before their eyes were they able, with his aid, to rise up from abject nothingness, poverty, terror.[5] In this view, the world's inhospitality—not to say hostility—toward human needs and wants arouses the disposition to self-help through technology.

By other accounts, the primary root is not weakness but strength: pride rather than needy fear erects the technological attitude. According to Genesis, for example, the first tool was the needle and the first artifact the fig leaf, when shame—which is here nothing but wounded pride—moved the primordial human beings to cover their nakedness, right from the moment of their rise to painful self-consciousness.[6] Pride lies behind the technological project of the city and tower of Babel, the human race being moved by the desire to make itself a name through artful self-assertion.[7] At the beginning of the modern era, Francis Bacon, himself moved by honor and glory, called mankind to the conquest of nature for the relief of man's estate, a project he regarded as the highest and most magnificent human possibility.[8] Ambition—the desire for wealth, power and honor—prompts many a man of science and industry. Finally, the master does not seek mastery just to escape from the cold.

There are, of course, other possible roots than fear, need and pride: for example, laziness, beneath the desire for an easier way to mow the lawn; boredom, beneath the desire for new amusements; greed, beneath the desire simply for more and more; vanity and lust, beneath the desire for new adornments and allurements; envy and hatred, beneath the desire to afflict those who make us feel low. And there is also the hard-to-describe desire to do something, to make something, to order something *just to see it done*—call it curiosity, call it willfulness, call it daring, call it perversity, call it will-to-power. I think we all know the motive, even from the inside.

This analysis of the origins of the technological disposition is, so far, only psychological, and goes deep into basic features of the human psyche. Yet this cannot be the whole story. For one thing, not all human societies would be rightly described as technological, even though all of them practice at least some of the arts. The people of ancient Israel and the Native Americans of the New World were not technological nations; neither is technology today the ruling outlook in Iran or in much of Africa. In place of the disposition to rational mastery, these societies and many others like them are ruled by the spirit of reverence, or national pride, or the passion for righteousness or holiness or nobility, or even just the intense devotion to one's own traditions. Even in the rationalist West, technological society seems to have appeared only in the last two centuries, and at its now runaway pace, only in the last seventy or eighty years. It certainly seems as if *modern* technology differs from ancient *techne*, not only in scale, but even, decisively, in its nature.

Whether or not this is so can be argued at length. But one thing is indisputable: modern technology would not be the ubiquitous phenomenon—or the problem—that it is, were it not for modern science, that daring and stupendous edifice of still-swelling knowledge, built only over the last 350 years, on foundations laid by Galileo, Bacon and Descartes. Says Robert Smith Woodbury in his article on the "History of Technology" for the *Encyclopaedia Britannica:* "For many thousands of years ... [man's] progress in technology was made by trial and error, by empirical advance.... It was only toward the end of the 18th century that technology began to become *applied science,* with results in the 19th and 20th centuries that have had enormous influence."⁹ A discussion of the nature of technology would be incomplete without at least a few words about modern science.

Though it is fashionable to distinguish *applied* from *pure* science—and it makes some sense to do so—it is important to grasp the essentially practical, social and technical character of modern science as such. Ancient science had sought knowledge of *what things are,* to be contemplated as an end in itself, satisfying to the knower. In contrast, modern science seeks knowledge of *how things work,* to be used as a means for the relief and comfort of *all humanity,* knowers and non-knowers alike. Though the benefits were at first slow in coming, this practical intention has been at the heart of modern science right from the start. Here, for example, is the celebrated announcement by Descartes of the good news of knowledge that is "very useful in life":

> So soon as I had acquired some general notions concerning Physics ... they caused me to see that it is possible to attain knowledge which is very useful in life, and that, instead of that speculative philosophy which is found in the Schools, we may find a *practical philosophy* by means of which, knowing the *force* and the *action* of fire, water, air, the stars, heaven, and all the other bodies that environ us, as distinctly as we know the different crafts of our artisans, we can in the same way *employ them* in all those uses *to which they are adapted,* and *thus render ourselves as the masters and possessors of nature.*¹⁰ [Emphasis added.]

But modern science is practical and artful not only in its ends. Its very notions and ways manifest a conception of the interrelation of knowledge and power. Nature herself is conceived energetically and mechanistically, and explanation of change is given in terms of (at most) efficient or moving causes; in modern science, to be *responsible* means to *produce an effect.* Knowledge itself is obtained productively: Hidden truths are gained by acting on nature, through experiment, twisting her arm to make her cough up her secrets. The so-called empirical science of nature is, as actually experienced, the highly contrived encounter with apparatus, measuring devices, pointer readings and numbers; nature in its ordinary course is virtually never directly encountered. Inquiry is made "methodical," through the imposition of order and schemes of measurement "made" by the intellect. Knowledge, embodied in *laws* rather than theorems, becomes "systematic" under rules of a new mathematics expressly *invented* for this purpose. This mathematics orders an "unnatural" world that has been intellectually "objectified," re-presented or pro-jected before the knowing subject as pure homogenous extension, ripe for the mind's grasping—just as the world itself will be grasped by the techniques that science will later provide. Even the modern word "concept" means "a grasping-together," implying that the mind itself, in its act of knowing, functions like the intervening hand—in contrast to its ancient counterpart, "idea," "that which can be beheld," which implies that the mind functions like the receiv-ing eye. And modern science rejects, as meaningless or useless, ques-tions that cannot be answered by the application of method. Science becomes not the representation and demonstration of truth, but an *art:* the art of finding the truth—or, rather, that portion of truth that lends itself to being artfully found. Finally, the truths that modern science finds—even about human beings—are value-neutral, in no way restraining technical application, and indeed perfectly adapted for it. In short, as Hans Jonas has put it, modern science contains manipulability at its theoretical core;[11] and this remains true even for those great scientists who are themselves motivated by the desire for truth and who have no interest in that mastery over nature to which their discoveries nonetheless contribute, and for which sci-ence is largely esteemed by the rest of us and mightily supported by the modern state.

For this reason, we must think of modern science and modern technology as a single, integrated phenomenon. It is the latter's fusion with the former that makes it both so successful and, as we shall see, such a problem.

## *What Is a Problem?*

If we now know what we might mean by "technology," we need also a few words about "problem" if we are fruitfully to address our question, "The Problem of Technology." What do we mean by "a problem"? This is no semantic game. For there is a deep difference between thinking of something as a problem and regarding it as, say, a question. (Heidegger's famous essay is "The *Question* Concerning Technology.") A "problem" (from the Greek *problema,* literally "something thrown out before" us) is any challenging obstacle, from a fence thrown up before an armed camp to a task set before someone to be done. Problems are publicly articulated tasks that challenge us to solve them, which is to say, to do away with them. When a problem is solved, it disappears; its solution is its *dissolution.* The solution is usually a construction, something we *make,* put together from elements into which the problem is broken up or, as we say, analyzed. We model the problem into a shape convenient for such analysis and construction; as we say, we *figure* it out. Further, a problem requires a solution *in its own terms;* the solution never carries one beyond the original problem as given.

The model of such problem solving is algebra. The equations containing unknowns are arranged, showing the analyzed elements in their constructed relations. The solutions that identify the unknowns dissolve the problem, and render the equation into an identity or tautology, which invites no further thought. But this mode of thought is not confined to algebra. It is the dominant mode of all modern scientific and technological thinking, in which, as we have seen, the mind makes its perplexities operational by turning them into problems that it can then methodically solve. But, further, this mode of thought is, in fact, the dominant mode of everyone's thinking much of the time. We are always trying to figure something out, to find a way over or around our obstacles, to solve our problems. We do not like to be obstructed, to be at a loss, to be resourceless. We do not like to have problems.

What, then, does it mean to treat technology as a problem, or to ask about *the* problem (or even the problems) of technology? For *whom* is technology an obstacle? More importantly, with respect to

*what goals* or desiderata does technology obstruct? Is it an obstacle to human happiness or to justice or to self-knowledge? Could
technology, understood as the disposition and activity of mastery,
turn out to be a stumbling block in the path of the master himself?
Finally, if technology is a problem, or poses a problem, what would
or could be its "solution"? If the difficulties caused by technology
are in fact only problems—say, for example, the problem of unintended side effects—we are certainly well advised to be looking for
solutions. But what if the difficulties attending technology are both
integral to its very being and inseparable from its benefits—like the
other side of a coin? This would make technology more like a tragedy
that begs for understanding and endurance, than like a problem that
calls for a solution. To put the point starkly: to formulate the question about technology as the *problem* of technology is itself a manifestation of technological thinking—of the desire to knock down
all obstacles, even if only in mind. To ask about the *problem* of technology in fact *exemplifies* it.

## The Problems of Technology

My warning about terminology notwithstanding, I am going to consider the problems of technology. Needless to say, I make no pretense of comprehensiveness. Moreover, I would not even attempt a
balance sheet of benefits and harms, even for a single circumscribed
technique; the task is virtually impossible, and the potential gain in
fundamental understanding slight. Finally, though I shall speak only
about problems—for clearly, the blessings of technology are well
known to us all—I am not, I repeat, an enemy of science and technology, at least in their proper measure, and I hold no brief for
romanticism, irrationality or the good old days. In those good old
days, most of us would very likely have either died in infancy or
spent our abbreviated life in arduous toil, and perhaps have been
persecuted for our heresies.

The first thing I would observe is that the argument about technology—or at least about the goodness and sufficiency of human
art and craftiness—is very old. Nearly everyone in antiquity agreed
that some form and degree of artfulness was indispensable for meeting

human needs and for human living together. No arts, no cities, and if no cities, no true humanity. Rational animal, technical animal, political animal—it is all one package. The arguments concerned rather the unqualified goodness of this package and, even more, the relative importance of *techne* and of law (or piety) in promoting the human good.

Crudely put, the argument could be stated this way. Those who hold that the biggest obstacles to human happiness are material, and arise from scarcity and the stinginess and violence of nature, from the indifference of the powers that be, or (within) from disease and death, look to the arts. In this view, the inventors and bringers of the arts are the true benefactors of mankind, and are revered like the gods; the supreme example is Prometheus (literally, "forethought"), bringer of fire, with its warming and transforming power, and through fire, all the other arts. By contrast, those who hold that the biggest obstacles to human happiness are psychic and spiritual, and arise from the turbulences of the human soul itself, look instead to law (or to piety or its equivalent) to tame and moderate the unruly and self-destroying passions of men. In this view, the lawgivers, the statesmen and the prophets are the true benefactors of mankind—not Prometheus but Lycurgus, not the builders of Babel but Moses. The arts are suspect precisely because they serve comfort and safety, because they stimulate unnecessary desires, and because they pretend to self-sufficiency. In the famous allegory of the cave in Plato's *Republic,* Socrates implies that it is the Promethean gift of fire and the enchantment of the arts that hold men unwittingly enchained, warm and comfortable yet blind to the world beyond the city. Mistaking their crafted world for the whole, men live ignorant of their true standing in the world and their absolute dependence on powers not of their own making and beyond their control.[12] Only when the arts and men are ruled politically, and only when politics is governed by wisdom about the human soul and man's place in the larger whole, can art contribute properly to human flourishing.

The coming of the modern technological project added a new wrinkle to this dispute. What if technology, founded upon the new science, could address not only stingy nature without but also unruly nature within? What if a science-based technology could be brought to bear on the human psyche (and human society) by means of a perfected psycho-physics (and scientific political science)? Might one then eventually secure human happiness by purely rational and technical means, without the need for law or force or fear of God? This was certainly part of the vision of Descartes, and, it seems, an anticipated benefit of the mastery of nature: "For the mind depends so much on the temperament and disposition of the bodily organs that, if it is possible to find a means of rendering men wiser and cleverer than they have hitherto been, I believe that it is in medicine that it must be sought."[13] Medicine, that venerable and most humanitarian of arts, will, when it is properly transformed by the new science of nature and human nature, provide at long last a solution for the human condition—through what we have only now begun to call biotechnology! (Later, after the Enlightenment, a similar promise was also tendered in the name of a scientific anthropology and sociology.)

### Feasibility

The first question arising from a consideration of the problems of modern technology is whether mastery of nature is feasible. Are we really *able* to exercise control, even over our material environment? Here we face first the practically important, though theoretically less interesting, problem of the unintended and undesired side effects of machine technology: air pollution, ozone depletion, soil erosion, acid rain, toxic wastes, nuclear fallout—a list of terribly serious problems, most of which can be remedied, if at all, only by more and better—not less—technology, including the techniques of monitoring and regulation. Even if the prophets of imminent ecological disaster exaggerate, theirs is an urgent cause. Indeed, Hans Jonas has powerfully argued that, thanks to the profound and global effects of twentieth-century technology, the whole scale and meaning of human action has been transformed, and a new ethic centered on responsibility for the entire earth needs urgently to be inculcated. Its new categorical imperative: "Do not compromise the conditions for an indefinite continuation of humanity on earth."[14]

Some consequences, called side effects because they are unwanted, are, in fact, not effects on the side. Intimately connected with the intended intervention, they must be seen, wanted or not, as *central* and integral to the whole. Consider automobility: by its very nature, it entails roads and bridges; the need for fuel and the dependence on oil; the rise of steel mills, auto factories, gas stations, garages, body shops, parking facilities and traffic laws; the production of noise, fumes, smog and auto graveyards; the need for autoworkers, auto dealers and mechanics, safety and highway inspectors, traffic police, parking attendants, driving instructors, testing and licensing personnel, insurance agents and claims adjusters, trackers of stolen cars, and medical personnel to deal with accidents and their human victims; and, thanks also to automobility itself, urban sprawl, homogenization through destruction of regional differences, separated lives for extended families, new modes of courtship behavior, new objects of envy and vanity, and a new battleground between parents and children appear quite predictably on the scene. Go assess and control the so-called unanticipated consequences of letting people rapidly move themselves about! Generally speaking, it is foolish to think that human beings can exercise extensive control over the consequences of technology, not least because the users' entire life can be altered in the process. As C. S. Lewis pointed out, we greatly exaggerate the increase in our power over nature that technology provides. In each generation, we bequeath to our descendants wonderful new devices, but by their aggregate effects, we preordain or at least greatly constrain how they are able to use them.[15]

More radical analysts of technology argue that modern technique is beyond human control *in principle*. Jacques Ellul, in his profound study *La Technique* (*The Technological Society*), argues that what looks like a free human choice between competing techniques is, in fact, *automatically* made, always in favor of greater efficiency; that technique encroaches everywhere, eliminating or transforming all previously nontechnical aspects of life; that technology augments itself irreversibly and in geometric progression; and that technology advances as if under an iron law: "Since it was possible, it was necessary."[16] This alleged automaticity of technology and its manifold effects, if true, would certainly embarrass the pretense to mastery. Winston Churchill put it starkly over fifty years ago, well before most of his contemporaries even suspected that there was any problem with technology:

Science bestowed immense new powers on man and, at the same time, created conditions which were largely beyond his comprehension and still more beyond his control. While he nursed the illusion of growing mastery and exulted in his new trappings he became the sport and presently the victim of tides and currents, whirlpools and tornadoes, amid which he was far more helpless than he had been for a long time.[17]

In this connection, let me just mention in passing the special kind of helplessness experienced by millions of people in the twentieth century as a result of modern despotism, to whose utopian programs and tyrannical successes and excesses modern technology—military, psychological, organizational, et cetera—contributed mightily. This sobering fact reminds us that what is called "man's power over nature" is, in fact, always power of some men over others—not only under despotisms but even when it is benevolently used. This thought about bad and good intentions leads us to the second problem, the problem of the *ends* of technology.

### Goals and Goodness

Let us set aside questions of feasibility and the problem of unwanted and unwelcome consequences, and think now only about the desired goals. What, on closer examination, can we say about the goals of the project for the mastery of nature?

As we have already noted, mastery of nature seeks, to begin with, man's liberation from chance and from natural necessity, both without and within: freedom from toil and lack, freedom from disease and depression, freedom from the risks of death. Put positively, these goals could be called comfortable sustenance, health (somatic and psychic) and longevity. Yet these wonderful things are not yet full human flourishing; providing the conditions for the pursuit of happiness, they are not happiness itself. Is there, in fact, any clear notion of happiness and human flourishing that informs the technological disposition?

Further, what is the *ground* of these and other goals? Where do they come from? Does liberation from natural necessity also mean liberation from natural goals? Or does man, even *qua* master of nature, remain within the grip of nature as regards his goals? Are not the goals of survival and pleasure, for example, given to man by his own nature? If so, then mastery over nature will always be incomplete: what looks like mastery will, in fact, be *service*—will be subordination to the dictates of nature spontaneously working within and finally beyond human control. Mastery will be enslavement to instincts, drives, lusts, impulsions, passions.[18]

On the other hand, perhaps technology can enable man to escape completely from the grip even of his own nature, even regarding the goals of mastery (though in another sense, of course, man cannot simply be outside of nature). If so, then mastery of nature would mean the virtually complete liberation of man *from nature's* control. Reason would not only be a tool, reason would create. Man would be free for full self-exertion, toward goals he freely sets for himself. Man's goals, like his means, would be his own projects. This alone would be genuine mastery, strictly speaking. (Something like this view of technology seems to be the understanding and the dream of Marxism.)

But what, one may then ask, would make these projects *good* and good *for us?* Why would the setting of projects by the untrammeled human will be anything but arbitrary? If we remember that man's so-called power over nature is, in truth, always a power exercised by some over others with knowledge of nature as their instrument, can it really be liberating to exchange the rule of nature for the rule of arbitrary human will? True, such will might happen to will philanthropically, but then again, and much more likely, it might not. If human history is any guide, we already know what to expect from the arbitrary positing of human projects, especially on a political scale. And even on a personal scale, is it really liberating—and fulfilling—to live under one's own will if that will, too, is arbitrary, if it takes no guidance from what would be genuinely good for oneself?

Fair enough, you say, but why must the mastering will be arbitrary? Why can't reason function not as an arbitrary creator, not merely as a tool, but also as a guiding eye, to discover and promulgate those standards of better and worse, right and good, justice and dignity, and true human flourishing that would guide the use of power and make the master not a capricious despot but a wise ruler? This is, of course, what all the nice people want and what they naively hope will happen. Indeed, the extreme trust in technology tacitly assumes the existence or the emergence of a kind of knowledge of genuine goals that would in fact guarantee not only the freedom but also the *goodness* of the mastery of nature.

Don't hold your breath. Such knowledge of goals and such standards for judging better and worse are not easily had, and they certainly cannot be provided by science itself. In the scientific view of the world, there can be no knowledge, properly speaking, about the purpose or meaning of human life, about human flourishing, or even about ethics: opinions about good and bad, justice and injustice, virtue and vice have no cognitive status and are not subject to rational inquiry. These, as we are fond of saying, are values, merely subjective. As scientists we can, of course, determine more or less accurately what it is different people *believe* to be good, but as scientists we are impotent to judge between them. Even political science, once the inquiry into how men *ought* to live communally, now studies only how they *do* live and the circumstances that move them to change their ways. Man's political and moral life is studied not the way it is lived, but abstractly and amorally, like a mere physical phenomenon.

The sciences are not only *methodologically* indifferent to questions of better and worse. Not surprisingly, they find their own indifference substantively reflected in the nature of things. Nature, as seen by our physicists, proceeds without purpose or direction, utterly silent on matters of better or worse, and without a hint of guidance regarding how we are to live. According to our biological science, nature is indifferent even as between health and disease; since both healthy and diseased processes obey equally and necessarily the same laws of physics and chemistry, biologists conclude that disease is just as natural as health. And concerning human longing, we are taught that everything humanly lovable is perishable, while all things truly eternal—like matter-energy or space—are utterly unlovable. The teachings of science, however gratifying as discoveries to the mind, throw icy waters on the human spirit.

Now science, in its neutrality to matters moral and metaphysical, can claim that it leaves to these separate domains the care of the good and matters of ultimate concern. This division of labor makes sense up to a point: Why should I cease to believe courage is good or murder is bad, just because science cannot corroborate these opinions? But this tolerant division of live and let live is intellectually unsatisfying and finally won't work. The teachings of science, as they diffuse through the community, do not stay quietly and innocently on the scientific side of the divide. They challenge and embarrass the notions about man, nature and the whole that lie at the heart of our traditional self-understanding and our moral and political teachings. The sciences not only fail to provide their own standards for human conduct; their findings cause us to doubt the truth and the ground of those standards we have held and, more or less, still tacitly hold.

The challenge goes much further than the notorious case of evolution versus biblical religion. Is there *any* elevated view of human life and goodness that is proof against the belief that man is just a collection of molecules, an accident on the stage of evolution, a freakish speck of mind in the mindless universe, fundamentally no different from other living—or even nonliving—things? What chance have the ideas of freedom and dignity, under even a high-minded *humanistic* dispensation, against the teachings of strict determinism in behavior and survival as the only natural concern of life? How fares the belief in the self-evident truths of the Declaration of Independence and the existence of inalienable rights to life, liberty and the pursuit of happiness, to whose defense the signers pledged their lives, their fortunes and their sacred honor? Does not the scientific worldview make us skeptical about the existence of *any* natural rights and therefore doubtful of the wisdom of those who risked their all to defend them? If survival and pleasure are the only possible principles that nature does not seem to reject, does not all courage and devotion to honor look like folly?

The chickens are coming home to roost. Liberal democracy, founded on a doctrine of human freedom and dignity, has as its most respected body of thought a teaching that has no room for freedom and dignity. Liberal democracy has reached a point, thanks in no small part to the success of the arts and sciences to which it is wedded, where it can no longer defend *intellectually* its founding principles. Likewise also the Enlightenment project, which has brought forth a science that can initiate human life in the laboratory yet cannot say what it means either by *life* or by *human*, a science whose teachings about man cannot even begin to support its own premise that enlightenment enriches life.

We are, quite frankly, adrift without a compass. We adhere more and more to the scientific view of nature and man, which both gives us enormous power and, at the same time, denies all possibility of standards to guide its use. Absent these standards we cannot judge our projects good or bad. We cannot even know whether progress is really progress or merely change—or, for that matter, decline.

### Tragic Self-Contradiction

Against these chilling thoughts, a small humanitarian voice protests that they are irrelevant. Surely, one does not need certain knowledge of the good to know the evils of human misery—of poverty, sickness, depression and death. Surely, much human good can be, has been and still will be accomplished by the effort to conquer them. Surely, it would be base to take lying down these beatings from stingy nature, and it can only be noble to rise up on our own behalf. These charges are surely right, as far as they go. But even this limited project for mastery is, *in principle*—that is, necessarily—doomed, not by its errors but by its very success. The master, simultaneously with his growing mastery—and as a result of it—also becomes more of a slave, not only through the unintended consequences of technology but from its victories. For the victories transform the souls and lives of the victors, preventing them from tasting triumph as success.

Consider, for example, the technology of meeting needs and relieving toil. We in the prosperous West have come a long way. But have we attained satisfaction? Have we not, with each new advance, seen our desires turn into needs, yesterday's luxuries into today's necessities? Thanks to human malleability, even need is an elastic notion, and human desires are, it seems, indefinitely inflatable. As desires swell and turn into needs, the gap between human want and satisfaction does not close, it grows wider.

Rousseau captured the point beautifully, describing the costs of even the first efforts at easing the harshness of life:

> [S]ince men enjoyed very great leisure, they used it to pursue many kinds of commodities unknown to their fathers; and that was the *first yoke* they imposed *upon themselves* without thinking about it, and the first source of the evils they prepared for their descendants. For, besides their continuing thus to soften body and mind, as these commodities had lost almost all their pleasantness through habit, and as they had at the same time *degenerated into true needs,* being deprived of them became much more cruel than possessing them was sweet; and people were unhappy to lose them *without being happy to have them.*[19] [Emphasis added.]

Moreover, new needs—especially in modern times—always create new dependencies, often on nameless and faceless others far away, on whose productivity and good will one comes increasingly to rely for one's own private happiness. Finally, since even poverty acquires only a relative meaning, since technology widens the possible range between rich and poor, since vanity and envy compound the gap and render it intolerable, satisfaction of need and desire becomes an ever-receding mirage. And should governments step in to try to level out the inequalities technology has spawned, they can do so only at the cost of economic liberty. Bureaucracy, too, is a form of technology, and living under it is anything but liberating. Does this look anything like mastery?

And what of technology fueled not by need but by fear of death? Has it proved a success? True, fear of death at the hands of wild animals rarely troubles the minds of city dwellers, but our haven against the animals has become a human jungle, where many walk—and dwell—in chronic fear of assault and battery, sometimes so enraged by their impotence to control the surrounding violence as to contribute to it themselves. On the international scene, we may credit the absence of fear of foreign invasion to our superior might, but the fear of death from modern warfare and international terrorism runs high, the unavoidable result of the fact that technologies know no political boundaries or that passenger airplanes can be used for more than transportation. Even in medicine, that heartland of gentle humanitarianism, the fear of death cannot be conquered. The greater our medical successes, the more unacceptable is failure and the more intolerable and frightening is death. True, many causes of death have been vanquished, but the fear of death has not abated, and may, indeed, have gotten worse. For as we have saved ourselves from the rapidly fatal illnesses, we now die slowly, painfully and in degradation—with cancer, AIDS or Alzheimer's disease. In our effort to control and rationalize death and dying, we have medicalized and institutionalized so much of the end of life as to produce what amounts to living death for thousands of people. Moreover, for these reasons we now face growing pressures for the legalization of euthanasia, which will complete the irony by casting the doctor, preserver of life, into the role of dispenser of death. We seem to be in the biomedical equivalent of a spiraling arms race with ourselves, creating technologies that heal only to cripple or crush, requiring us to respond either by seeking more technologies that heal or by electing a technological escape from life altogether. Does this sound like mastery?

Finally, what of those technologies for the soul, only now being marshaled, to combat depression and dementia, stress and schizophrenia? What of applied psychology and neurochemistry, behavior modification and psychopharmacology? If modern life contributes mightily to unhappiness, can we not bring technology to the rescue? Can we not make good on the Cartesian promise to make men stronger and better in mind and in heart, by understanding the material basis of aggression, desire, grief, pain and pleasure? Would this not be the noblest form of mastery, the production of artful self-command, without the need for self-sacrifice and self-restraint? On the contrary. Here the final technical conquest of his own nature would almost certainly leave mankind utterly enfeebled. This form of mastery would be identical with utter dehumanization. Read Huxley's *Brave New World,* read C. S. Lewis's *Abolition of Man,* read Nietzsche's account of the last man, and then read the newspapers. Homogenization, mediocrity, pacification, drug-induced contentment, debasement of taste, souls without loves and longings—these are the inevitable results of making the essence of human nature the last project for technical mastery. In his moment of triumph, Promethean man will become also a contented cow.

Having enumerated a number of problems of technology, can we find their common ground? What shall we say is *the* problem of technology? I would suggest that "the problem of technology" is that technology is not problem but tragedy, the poignantly human adventure of living in grand self-contradiction. In tragedy the failure is imbedded in the hero's success, the defeats in his victories, the miseries in his glory. The technological way, deeply rooted in the human soul and spurred on by the utopian promises of modern thought, seems to be inevitable, heroic and doomed.

To say that technology as a way of life is doomed, left to itself, does not yet mean that modern life—*our* life—*must* be tragic. Everything depends on whether the technological disposition is allowed to proceed to its self-augmenting limits, or whether it can be resisted, spiritually, morally, politically.

## *Technology and Liberal Democracy*

Many Americans today—including, one should emphasize, the critics as well as the friends of technology—share, explicitly or tacitly, the rationalist's dream of human perfectibility. But the Founders of the American Republic, though influenced by optimistic Enlightenment thought, were hardly utopians. They adopted a more moderate course. On the one hand, they knew human nature well enough not to underestimate the crucial importance of good laws (backed by enforcement), education and also religion for the preservation of decency and public spiritedness. On the other hand, they appreciated fully the promise of science. The American Republic is, to my knowledge, the first regime explicitly to embrace scientific and technical progress and to claim its importance for the public good. The United States Constitution, which is silent on education and morality, speaks up about scientific progress:

> The Congress shall have power ... To promote the Progress of Science and useful Arts, by securing for limited Times to Authors and Inventors the exclusive Right to their respective Writings and Discoveries. (Article I, Section 8)

Our Founders, in this singular American innovation, encouraged technological progress by adding the fuel of interest to the fire of genius.

Yet progress for progress's sake was not their goal. Rather, by science and technology they hoped to help provide for the common defense, promote the general welfare and, above all, secure the blessings of *liberty* to ourselves and our posterity.

Given liberal democracy's devotion to liberty and equality, it should be no surprise that liberal democracy stands in an uneasy and mixed relationship to the technological project. On the one hand, it provides the perfect soil for technological growth. Economic and personal freedom, the emancipation of inventiveness and enterprise, the restless striving for improvement, the absence of class barriers to personal ambition, and the (fortuitous) natural wealth and expanse of our particular land have given technology perhaps the most hospitable home it has ever had. Moreover, the preservation of our liberties, no less than our general welfare, have been tied on more than one occasion to American engineering, rational planning and methodical social organization—I refer in particular to the Second World War. As our liberal democracy becomes also a mass society, with mass culture, bureaucratization, multinational corporations, big government, and so on, our need for and infatuation with technology increases, not only in terms of equipment but also in efforts to rationalize and administer all economic and social arrangements. If we add to this our American individualism, materialism, acquisitiveness, and all the other democratic traits so well described by Tocqueville, we see clearly the danger of the intensification of all the problems of technology, as we cheerfully race our engines toward (at best) the soft and dehumanized despotism of Brave New World.

At the same time, however, American liberal democracy, rightly understood, also contains some seeds of a possible remedy for the problem of technology, or rather for remembering that the problem with technology stems from embracing its vision wholeheartedly. We liberal democrats may not be able to stem the technological tide, but we do have the wherewithal to keep from going under. Everything depends on rejecting the rationalist and utopian dream of perfecting human beings by re-creating them, and on remembering that richer vision of human liberty and human dignity that informs the founding of our polity.

I point to three aspects of that vision. First, liberty means political liberty. It means self-rule, not self-indulgence. It means participating in local government and community affairs, not demanding government benefits. It means not only exercising rights and making claims, but being willing to defend those rights, with one's life and fortune and sacred honor if necessary. The American citizen is not a happy slave. True, prospects for active citizenship today often seem greatly attenuated, thanks largely to changes of scale and governance for which technology is largely responsible: it is not clear what citizenship means or requires in the megalopolis or in the superbureaucratic state. Yet voluntary associations abound, many with civic and public-spirited purpose; and the liberation from arduous toil brought by technology affords many more people sufficient leisure to get involved—in schools, neighborhood organizations, local politics and countless philanthropic and civic-minded activities.

Political liberty also allows for genuine political deliberation and action. The people's representatives are capable of responding to the problems spawned by technology, from enacting standards for the purity of air and water, to preserving natural forests and parks against the deadening encroachments of asphalt. In the biomedical area, the same Congress that enacted the patent laws also established the Food and Drug Administration, mandated the creation of institutional review boards (IRBs) to protect human subjects of biomedical research, and outlawed the buying and selling of organs for transplantation. Various states have enacted legislation prohibiting assisted suicide, destructive research on embryos, and cloning. As this book goes to press, the United States Senate is poised to debate a national ban on all human cloning, the House of Representatives having passed such a ban in July 2001. If we have the political will, American institutions offer us political opportunities to redirect, regulate and slow down the technological juggernaut.

Second, liberty means the freedom of private life, a domain of "real life" rather than virtual reality. Homes, families, friends, parents and children dwell in a realm of sentiment and spontaneous affection, rooted in the bonds of lineage and relation, and presided over by some of the deepest strengths of our nature. Private life is where we come face to face with birth and love, death and sorrow, not merely as helpless victims but as connected, responsible and thoughtful agents. Private life also provides liberty of worship, to acknowledge the dependence of human life—and of nature itself—on powers beyond us and not at our disposal. Technology today threatens our private life by invading our houses to make us, in effect, comfortably homeless. Television usurps the place of conversation, while modern conveniences diminish time spent cooperatively meeting necessity. The contraceptively liberated discover sadly that pursuit of easy gratification rarely leads to deep and enduring intimacy. Marriages and families are notoriously unstable and children suffer, often in the midst of extraordinary advantages and opportunities. But at the same time, we increasingly know what we are missing; people are learning that marriages and friendships need their sustained attention, and there is renewed interest in religion among the young, one suspects because of their dissatisfaction with a merely technical orientation toward life. As long as families and religious bodies affirm their essentially nontechnical dispositions in the world, a remedy against dehumanization may still be found.

Finally, liberalism means liberal education. Not just education for employment or even for citizenship, important though these are, but education for thoughtfulness and understanding, in search of genuine wisdom. Full human dignity requires a mind uncontaminated by ideologies and prejudice, turned loose from the shadows of the cave, free not only to solve factitious problems of its own devising, but free to think deeply about the meaning of human existence and, especially in a world overshadowed by technology, to think about the nature and purpose and goodness of science and technology. If the deepest problem of technology lies in the narrowly utilitarian habit of mind it engenders, liberal education offers an antidote. In liberal democracy, and especially in liberal education, lies the last best hope of mankind.

Honesty compels me to add, straightaway, that liberal education—like both active citizenship and rich private life—is not flourishing in American society. In our colleges and universities, genuinely liberal learning is sacrificed to preoccupations with narrow specialization, vocational and technological training, trendy intellectual fashions, ideological disputes and indoctrination, and just plain foolishness and frivolity. Yet nearly everywhere, one can find pockets of thoughtfulness and genuine inquiry—a sound program here, a superb teacher or two there—beacons of light that attract and engage serious and eager students. It has been my singular good fortune to be first a student and then for twenty-five years a teacher in one such pocket, the College of the University of Chicago, whose ethos has encouraged teachers and students alike to think deeply about the most important human matters. Unlike the inhabitants of Brave New World, we are still free and able to swim intellectually against the technocratic tide, preserving in our souls a place for the glory of genuine thought and the quest for truth and meaning.

In the end, however, the freedom of private life and the power of democratic political institutions will be no better than the moral character of the people and the ethical norms they revere and embody. And liberal education, beautiful jewel that it is, cannot alone provide the moral foundations of a community once they are eroded, nor can it, by itself, produce patriotic citizens, honorable fathers and mothers, or even decent neighbors. As I will argue in the next chapter, "expert" professors of ethics or bioethics are likewise unequal to these tasks. They are tasks, rather, for families and for communities of worship, where cultural practices enable the deepest insights of the mind to become embodied in the finest habits of the heart. Not for nothing does the Good Book say that the beginning of wisdom is the "fear [awe, reverence] of the Lord."

# CHAPTER TWO

# Practicing Ethics:
# Where's the Action?

*I had sooner play cards against a man who was quite skeptical about
ethics, but bred to believe that "a gentleman does not cheat," than
against an irreproachable moral philosopher who had been brought up
among sharpers.* —C. S. Lewis, The Abolition of Man

When I first took up questions of bioethics over thirty
years ago, I was a young biochemist working at
the National Institutes of Health, researching problems that had
solutions, albeit about bacterial physiology. Today I guess I would
call myself an aging humanist, pursuing questions without final
answers about human nature and human good, and I can boast only
of having at last become old enough to be entitled to my somewhat
traditional beliefs and concerns. One conclusion I have reached is
that the field of bioethics has also grown older these past thirty years,
but, if I may say so, not especially wiser.

Since our concern here is with the present and the future, we
will not indulge in nostalgia. Still, it is useful to remind ourselves of
a few salient facts. First, the late 1960s were a turbulent time for
American society, but a sleepy time for the study of ethics. Academic
philosophy busied itself with other things, and no one had ever heard
of "ethicists." Second, the effects of the so-called biological revolution were only just beginning to be felt: oral contraceptives and psy-
chedelic drugs were in use and the first heart transplant had just been
performed, but legal abortion, fetal tissue implantation, prenatal
genetic diagnosis, human *in vitro* fertilization and embryo transfer,
surrogate motherhood, stem cell research, pre-implantation genetic
diagnosis, gene synthesis and gene therapy, Prozac, brain implants,

hospices, and "Do Not Resuscitate" orders were things of the future, though some of them were already foreseeable. Third, those of us who gathered to found the first American think tank for bioethics (The Hastings Center), though we came from a variety of cultural and professional backgrounds, shared a concern for the human meaning of these and other anticipated new biomedical developments. Some of us inclined toward hope, eager to have the benefits of new technologies, but with protections against error and folly. Others of us inclined toward fear, repelled by certain prospects of biomedical intervention and concerned that even the well-intentioned uses of the new powers over the human body and mind might inadvertently diminish our humanity. But although we were moved variously, moved all of us were by moral or religious sentiments and concerns. All of us understood that the new biomedical technologies touched—and perhaps threatened—fundamental aspects of what it means to be a human being. If I remember correctly, only one of the founding fellows of the Hastings Center made his living teaching philosophy, and he would come to meetings only if they did not require that he violate the Sabbath. It goes without saying, but it is important to note, that none of us *came into* bioethics through either the study or the practice of bioethics as it is now practiced and studied.

That was then. This is now and the ethics business is booming. There is ethics action everywhere. Most medical schools offer courses in medical ethics; in colleges and universities undergraduate ethics courses abound; and some philosophy departments offer doctorates in bioethics. There are numerous journals of bioethics and a national professional society that accredits members of the guild. Many hospitals have established ethics committees, mainly but not exclusively for dealing with decisions regarding termination of treatment, while institutional review boards must rule on all sorts of experimentation with human subjects. Courts of law are increasingly asked to settle ethical conflicts, while blue ribbon commissions, national and local, analyze issues and formulate guidelines to govern practice. Many other research institutes have followed the Hastings Center into the field, and the literature—professional and popular—grows, it seems, exponentially. And ethicists are in vogue: they get positions in medical schools, are quoted in the daily papers on every hot topic, and appear frequently on television and radio talk shows. Many of them are even in the employ of the biotechnology companies, serving as in-house advisors who pronounce ethical blessings on the latest innovations. In one generation, biomedical ethics has become not only established, but also part of the establishment. Bioethics is where the action is.

Yet it is far from clear that we have cause for celebration. The rise of professional bioethics may have been good for bioethicists, but how good has it been for our ethics? Have there been substantial improvements in the practices and moral sensibilities of physicians, scientists, entrepreneurs, or the general public in matters ethical or bioethical? Are the choices that we are making, individually or socially, regarding the development and use of the awesome powers biology is providing us better than they were thirty years ago and better than they would have been in the absence of the work of bioethicists? How effective is the practice of ethics now?

## *Practicing Ethics Today*

In bioethics at present, the action is mostly talk. By itself, this is not surprising, for to act as a human being often means deliberating and consulting beforehand, in search of what best to do. But the language of ethicists is not generally that of moral agents faced with the necessity for action. Even when we consider specific cases or actions, our talk is frequently abstract and theoretical. In fact, much of the practice of ethics these days is really *meta*-ethical. It seeks to analyze and clarify moral argumentation; to establish or criticize grounds for justifying our decisions; to lay down rules and guidelines, principles and procedures, for addressing ethical dilemmas; and, in some cases, to construct comprehensive theories of conduct centering around fundamental norms, called "autonomy" or "utility" or "duty" or "equality" or "beneficence."

An example may help illuminate the difference between real moral deliberation and abstract bioethics talk. An elderly woman, once proudly strong and independent but now moderately demented and in a nursing home, has spoken for several years of her desire to die. In fact, she has regularly asked her son for poison to help her take her own life—requests he has sympathetically heard but steadfastly refused. One day the woman suffers a stroke and, on top of it, develops double pneumonia. The nursing home physician recommends hospitalization and antibiotics. Mindful of the woman's reiterated wish to die and her new disabilities from the stroke, several family members oppose treating her pneumonia (a disease that, before the age of antibiotics, used to be called "the old man's friend"). But her physician, a man who sees himself as servant of the patient's good and who regards it as immoral not to treat reversible life-threatening infections, is adamant. Intense conversation ensues about the possible and probable consequences of both action and inaction. Despite their differences of opinion, however, everyone involved is animated by the same goal: trying to figure out what is really best for this particular woman here and now, in light of all that is known about her history, circumstances, prospects and expressed wishes.

The patient herself is, owing to the stroke and fever, less responsive than usual, and she says little in reply to the doctor's direct questioning. But her son, who knows from long experience how best to reach and read his mother, persists in trying to get through to her. Putting questions in a variety of different ways, he finally manages to get her to see what needs to be decided and that she has a choice. "You have bad pneumonia," he tells her, "and the doctor thinks you should go to the hospital. But you don't have to go if you don't want to." "Well," mumbles the elderly woman to the family's surprise, "if they can make me feel a little bit better, I'll go (to the hospital)." The matter is settled. The well-meaning family is prevented from electing death for the patient who, when talk of death comes to action, is not really eager to surrender.

More often than not these days, individual human dramas such as this are resolved not by the principal agents but by referral to hospital ethicists or ethics committees. The discussions there, very different from the ones near the bedside, are generalized, remote, highly influenced by the current fashions of bioethics. The ethicists have their profession's own terms of analysis; the committees have their rules of procedure and decision making. Incapable of genuine and intimate knowledge of the patient, both ethicist and committee would necessarily treat her as but a generic instance of her class: a demented woman in a nursing home who has often and clearly expressed a wish to die, but who now is incapable of making the choice to do so. In place of the engaged familial concern for the well-being of a loved one at the end of her long life, we get a shrunken discussion framed as a particular instance of the so-called "termination of treatment" problem.

Arguments will be made about "medical paternalism," the charge that doctors wrongfully exercise a tyranny of expertise over moral decisions that rightly belong to the patient. The principle of "patient autonomy" (the supremacy of the right to choose) will be asserted against the principle of "beneficence" (the obligation to do good and to avoid harm). Meta-ethical arguments will be made about whether the right moral theory here should be "consequentialist" (weighing benefits versus harms) or "deontological" (doing one's duty to what is right, regardless of the consequences). There will be debates about the nature and utility of the distinction between *ordinary* and *extraordinary* means of saving life, and whether antibiotics in this instance constitute one or the other. There will be disputes about whether there is a difference between "allowing to die" and "deliberately killing," or whether declining to offer antibiotics amounts to assisted suicide. There will be inquiry about the existence of a "living will" or of patient-directed "orders not to resuscitate," and, in the absence of such evidence, much will be made of the woman's oft-expressed request for assistance in suicide.

Although a generalized fear of a lawsuit shadows the hospital's ethics committee, its members will take up the case in relation to "a right to death with dignity" or "a right to die," ideas that are custom-made for litigation.* When such matters do reach the courts, there is no limit to the mischief that ethical theory can do. Sophistic arguments are offered not only in defense of "a right to die" but also in the name of theories of justice or equality: for example, "it is *inherently unfair* that patients on dialysis or respirators can elect death by shutting off the machines, while this elderly woman is denied a wished-for death via physician-assisted suicide and must therefore now suffer further debility and disgrace." In many cases, the abstract principle of autonomy or equality, asserted seemingly on the patient's behalf, will win the day, but to the neglect of the individual patient herself. Her concrete human situation is drowned out by a flood of theory. And the result can be deadly.

---

*These notions will be discussed at length in Chapters Seven and Eight.

Faced with all this ethics talk and theory, one may well wonder, "Where's the action?" What is the connection between this practice of ethical *discourse,* now vigorously conducted by ethicists and their collaborators, and ethical *practice,* that is, the deeds of medical practitioners, hospital administrators, public health officials, and the countless citizens who have dealings with them?

I come to this matter in a moment, but first let me describe in greater detail what I regard as some of the dominant fashions in the practice of ethics now flourishing. These generalizations do not apply to all practitioners today, but they seem to me to characterize both the mainstream and its most prominent navigators.

First, ethics is seen first and foremost as a field of *theorizing.* Though ethics is eventually concerned with matters of conduct — with what we do and how we live — most scholars of ethics are theorists, who do not begin concretely with real actors and deeds but abstractly with ideas about action and its proper justifications. Dealing with action is thought to be *applying* theory to practice, like applied science or engineering.

Second, as theory, ethics today belongs in particular to *philosophical* theorizing. To practice ethics means especially to practice the academic discipline of philosophical ethics. To be sure, the field is home also to people who call themselves religious ethicists, even Christian or Jewish ethicists, but most of these use the terminology and play by the rules laid down by academic philosophy. Religious thought — I would hesitate to call it theorizing — has its own profound understanding of the human condition and teachings about the moral life, an understanding deep enough to help us address the large questions of our humanity at stake in life's encounters with biotechnology. But the pluralistic premises of American ethical discourse and the fashions of the modern academy lead the mainstream to view such religious traditions at best with suspicion and often with outright contempt. Even religious ethicists seem to accept this judgment — the late Paul Ramsey being a most notable exception.* Perhaps for the sake of getting a broader hearing, perhaps so as not to

---

*Ramsey, for many years professor of Christian ethics at Princeton University, was one of the intellectual founders of the modern study of bioethics. His pioneering works, *The Patient As Person* and *Fabricated Man*, both published in 1970, remain classics

profane sacred teachings or in order to preserve a separation between the things of Caesar and the things of God, or perhaps from sheer embarrassment over their religious attachments, most religious ethicists entering the public practice of ethics leave their special religious insights at the door and talk about "deontological vs. consequentialist," "autonomy vs. paternalism," "justice vs. utility," just like everybody else.

Third, philosophical ethics today is *rationalist,* I would say "*hyper*-rational," and, I would allege, unreasonably so. The dominant mode of American philosophizing today remains analytic. It concerns itself with the analysis of concepts, the evaluation of arguments and the criticism of justifications, always in search of clarity, consistency, coherence. It spends little time on what genuinely moves people to act—their motives and passions: that is, loves and hates, hopes and fears, pride and prejudice, matters that are sometimes dismissed as nonethical or irrational because they are not simply reducible to *logos.* Revulsions and their correlative taboos are also overlooked; since they cannot give incontrovertible logical defenses of themselves, they tend to fall beneath the floor of ethical discourse. As a result, that discourse focuses almost exclusively on matters conceptual and logical.

In substance no less than in form, the ethics mainstream tends to be rationalist. The supreme focus of moral concern is not *human beings* as needy and aspiring, embodied souls (or enlivened bodies) enmeshed in formative relations with other human beings, but "*personhood,*"—the independent rational will or the conscious subject. Personhood becomes the touchstone of our dignity because it is the ground of our autonomy. Reason finds reasons to defend the citadel of rationality alone.

Fourth, as we saw in the last chapter, rationality at work is above all a *problem solver.* As in science, so in ethics, rationality's first task is to define and isolate some matter of human concern as a problem demanding or seeking solution. Intelligibility and clarity are purchased at the cost of abstraction, and frequently also of

---

in the field. Though I never shared his religious starting points, my own early education in bioethics owes much to the instruction and friendship of this outstanding thinker and man of moral principle.

distortion. For example, out of the poignant and complicated human situations surrounding the end of life, filled with the difficulties of facing death and caring for the dying, we isolate as a separate problem "When to pull the plug?" or "Can a physician morally hasten the end of life?" Out of the deeply significant relations between parents and children, we isolate as a problem to be solved the legitimacy of contracts for surrogate pregnancy or the ownership of laboratory-preserved human embryos. Out of the AIDS epidemic, we isolate a problem of privacy versus public safety, or we treat the whole matter as a problem whose solution is a new drug or a better condom. In each of these cases, when we "find a problem" we also abstract it from its meaning in relation to human intimacy, trust, fidelity, moderation, and moral and sexual responsibility.

A problem, once it has been abstracted as a problem, is also abstractly analyzed. To be sure, these analyses are often interesting, but because of their rationalistic cast they rarely follow the lines of deliberation followed by prudent agents faced with the need to act. As we saw with the earlier example, choosing the best course of action, in light of the concrete circumstances, is not the same thing as analyzing and solving a formulated problem pulled out of context. Not only does the rationalist analysis fail to reach desires and goals, motives and ends. It also often neglects the normative questions of which ends are to be preferred, here and now. (I note in passing a serious danger in ethics seen as rational problem solving: such an ethics does not fill the human void created by technological thinking, nor does it supply the fully human response to the need to act. Rather, rationalistic ethics becomes merely a countervailing technique, the ethicist another technical expert like the ophthalmologist or the cardiologist, in danger of being a specialist without vision and a moralist without heart.)

Fifth, in its penchant for setting and solving problems, today's approach to ethics abstracts still further from the rich context of our moral life by concentrating mainly on the *extreme examples*. The implantation of an artificial (or chimpanzee) heart or the use of surrogate wombs or the definition of death or guidelines for terminating life-sustaining treatment capture most of the attention—not surprisingly—but the morality of ordinary practice is largely ignored. Yet every human encounter is an ethical encounter, an occasion for the practice (and cultivation) of virtue and respect, and, between doctors and patients, for the exercise of responsibility and trust, on both sides. How do physicians speak to patients? Do they respect and protect their privacy and vulnerabilities? Do patients have reasonable expectations of their physicians? How do we, individually and culturally, stand with respect to rearing children, sharing intimacies, revering life, facing death? In the absence of attention to these more fundamental and pervasive moral postures and practices, is it reasonable to expect that an ethics for the extreme cases will be sensibly worked out even in theory, let alone be successful when "applied" to practice?

Sixth, when rational problem solving solves its ethical problems, the solutions themselves tend to be purely rational, often taking the form either of rules or of ideals—rational *rules* that should govern conduct; articulable *ideals* toward which practice should strive. Not addressed are moral sensibilities and affections or habits and customs of moral agents. Moreover, as rational, rules and ideals tend to be enunciated as universals, with no attention paid to the necessary particularity of judgment that all moral action involves.

Sometimes rational problem solving, mindful of cultural pluralism and personal differences, draws back from offering substantive rules or ideals. Instead, rational *procedures* for making decisions are devised, without any attempt to specify the content of the decisions that will be duly made. There is no question that establishing guidelines for the termination of treatment, for example, can alert decision makers to otherwise neglected considerations, especially where the situation calling for action occurs under conditions of emotional distress. Yet, here too, universalized and abstract procedures are proposed without attention to customary practices or previously existing patterns for seeking advice, making choices, or living with the ambiguity of the choices made. No guidelines can cover all real cases, much less touch the critical nuances that distinguish any one case from another. The methodical rationality of procedure is put in place of the discerning reasonableness of the prudent man-on-the-spot that all real choices demand.

Finally, the rationalistic devotion to moral ideals leads moral thought in the direction of *ideology,* always many steps removed from moral life as lived. Some moral theorists focus largely on solving "systemic problems" rather than, say, on improving the moral conduct of individual agents. For example, one recent commentator, complaining about the screening of employees for illegal drug use, decries "our penchant to focus on individual citizens instead of systemic social problems. We seem to think that by treating citizens like grapes from Chile to be screened for cyanide ... we can solve our problems of poverty, racism, and violence." But do these social evils exempt individuals from the responsibility to be in their right drug-free minds if they are to drive school buses or control air traffic? And how do the "systemic problem fixers" expect a society to fight poverty, racism, and violence in the abstract, especially if it is indifferent to the concrete moral well-being and vigor of its particular citizens? Conversely, other theorists make an ideology out of "autonomy," without regard to the content of choices freely made, but, curiously, show no concern with the social institutions and communal mores that nurture the growth of self-determining adults and that guide their every choice and deed. For example, some bioethicists reject any restrictions on the practices of surrogate pregnancy or even human cloning, all in the name of the freedom to choose or the freedom to reproduce, by whatever means. These ideals turned into ideologies may effectively dramatize weaknesses and shortcomings in existing practices, but because of their abstractness they are powerless to form new customs and practices. And, as the idealized best is frequently the enemy of the actual good, ideologies, sometimes inadvertently, help dismantle the living and habitual moral fabric of a society that, alone, can help reform existing conduct.

I know that this crude sketch of the practice of ethics is at best incomplete and suffers from, among other things, *my own* predilections toward abstraction and generalization. And despite my criticism of this approach to ethics—soon to be made more explicit—I do not underestimate its contributions. Thanks to the work of the last three decades, consciousness has been raised, moral complacency and indifference to moral matters have been partly overcome, some issues have been clarified, some thoughtless and unreasonable prejudices have been countered, competing goods have been identified and to some degree balanced, and, in general, ethically troublesome situations are faced more deliberately and self-consciously—though, in my view, not obviously with wiser choices or finer deeds or better outcomes. At least until now, the field of medical ethics and bioethics has attracted (if we may say so ourselves) a rather high-minded and principled group of scholars and teachers—no Jimmy Swaggarts and Al Sharptons in our parish. The earnestness of many of the practitioners and the sobriety of their speech seems to be promoting a more reflective and reasonable approach, at least among those who participate in the colloquies. And the elaboration of procedures and guidelines and the institution of committee decision making have had perhaps the secondary benefit of promoting community of discourse, again, among those who participate.

Yet, as I have already hinted, this theoretical and rationalistic approach to ethics has grave weaknesses. It speaks little about motives and attitudes, and still less about how to get people to do what theory says is best. Universalist in conception, it cares little for the variety of human types, some moved by the love of gain, others by the love of honor, some by reverence, others by fear, still others by pleasure. In short, it treats the rational content of speech and argument without regard to the engaged concerns that incite both speech and action. It by and large ignores mores and customs, sentiments and attitudes, and the "small morals" that are the bedrock of ordinary experience and the matrix of all interpersonal relations. It by and large ignores real moral agents and concrete moral situations, preferring the abstraction of the hypostasized "rational decision maker" confronting the idealized problem needing to be solved. Because real life is too complicated, it frequently prefers its own far-out, cleverly contrived dilemmas, for example, thinking about abortion by conjuring a woman who wakes up to find a world-famous violinist grafted onto her body. Regarding the deeper matters and ultimate human concerns that lie just beneath the surface of everyday life—the significance of human finitude or the moral worth of suffering or the meaning of sexuality and procreation—it has virtually nothing to say. Of the rich broth of our social-civil-cultural-spiritual life together, and of the ways in which it seasons us all without our knowing it, we theoreticians know almost nothing. Though originally intended to improve our deeds, the reigning practice of ethics, if truth be told, has, at best, improved our speech.

## Theory and Practice: Speech and Deed

Is this a fair charge? It is difficult to know. We would need to assess comprehensively whether and how the rise of the practice of ethics as theory has been beneficial for ethical practice in action. Such an assessment is beyond my powers. But those of us who entered the field concerned about the road leading to *Brave New World* cannot be reassured. Some of the worrisome or repugnant biomedical technologies (for example, extracorporeal conception and surrogate motherhood; sex selection; perfusion of newly dead bodies as "organ farms"; pre-implantation genetic selection) have begun to arrive and are being used—to be sure, all with "suitable guidelines," and with the appropriate chorus of earnest concern about possible misuses and moral costs. Bioethicists have by and large behaved as if they could (and should) do no more than give pious blessings to the inevitable; and those who are now employed by the biotech companies whose activities they ought to be scrutinizing are even being rewarded for not rocking the boat.

And what about the institutions in which medicine is practiced: do they treat people, humanly speaking, any better than they did thirty years ago? Are hospital staffs more civil and engaged? Are nurses and doctors listening and speaking better with patients? Have our required courses and conferences on medical ethics improved the characters and mores of our rising physicians? They may now be prepared to write "Do Not Resuscitate" orders, but does their new sensitivity to last things stop there? Are they better at attending the dying *before* the occasion of cardiac arrest? And what of their general manners and sensibilities? In my family's and my students' own recent experiences with physicians and hospitals, the following incidents give pause: emergency-room physicians, one after the next, fail to introduce themselves; gynecologists (and their nurses) refer to patients only by first names and conclude their consultations while the women are still lying undressed on the examining tables; a professor of pediatrics displays an intelligent ten-year-old child with a genetic abnormality, telling the class in the child's presence that had he been conceived today he would have been aborted; a group of (male and female) doctors and medical students stand around the bed discussing its occupant, oblivious to his profound discomfort at being left there stark naked and uncovered (a distressed medical student who later complained to her professor about these last two incidents was told that she was too sensitive for the practice of medicine); an intern greets the ambulance in which I am riding bringing my mother to the hospital by screaming at the paramedics because proper telephone notification had not been given; the attending physician on call for his group practice refuses to accept calls except in an emergency.

What sorts of people are being selected for medicine and from whom are they learning what about its ordinary decent and humane practice?

More generally, what has ethical theory been able to do for the malpractice crisis, itself a cause and a symptom of a massive breakdown of trust, or for the consequences of the new economic forces operating in medicine? Or again, for all our talk about reproductive ethics, are our families more stable and stronger today? For all our talk about death and dying, are our elderly parents better cared for by us than were their parents by them? Most generally, what about those forces of moral education in the popular culture—music, movies, television? Have they reached a higher standard of decency and moral taste? Will it be said of us that we ethicists fine-tuned our theoretical fiddles while modern Rome rocked and rolled its way back to barbarism?

These are, of course, all large and empirical questions, and I raise them here not so much to seek answers as to hammer home the question about theory and practice. Even if one could prove cultural and professional moral decline or standstill during our rebirth of theorizing, that would not necessarily be theory's fault. No one in biomedical ethics promised to work miracles. But our reigning theory can, I think, be faulted for its insufficient and faulty attention precisely to this matter of the relation between moral theory and moral action.

How does one get from theory to practice, from speech to deed, according to current theory? *Application* is said to be the way, as in "applied ethics." "To apply," from the Latin *applicare,* means to bring into direct contact, to lay upon, to lean against. To apply a theory (or a rule or a rational principle) means bringing it, from the outside, into direct contact with . . . with what? Why, with a moral agent, and presumably with his desires or motives or will, with whatever is the mainspring of his action. But does anybody consider why the motive should care to listen to the applied speech, why appetite should allow itself to be influenced by the applied rules or ideals? As Aristotle noted long ago, thought—or speech or reason—itself *moves nothing*, especially, one can add, thought merely laid down *next to* appetite. Thought, to be effective, must be *inseparable* from appetite.*

The true source of action is not abstract thought, nor even thought *applied* to some separate motor or motive force, but rather a concretion, a grown-togetherness, of appetite and mind, so intertwined that one cannot say for sure whether the human principle of action is a species of desire become thoughtful, or an activity of intellection suffused with appetite. How mind and desire become grown together is, of course, a great question, but it is rarely accomplished by applying purely rational doctrines or rules in a passionless way to human agents. On the contrary, the true beginning is rather with the direct but unreflective education of our loves and hates, our pleasures and pains, gained only in practice, through habituation and by means of praise and blame, reward and punishment. Anyone concerned with influencing conduct must be concerned with these in-between powers of the soul, themselves irrational (in the sense of nonreasoning) but fully amenable to reason (in the sense of being formed, to begin with, in accordance with the reasons of one's parents, teachers and laws, and being open to further refinement through the exercise of one's own powers of deliberation and discernment).

In short, our current concept of the relation of theory to practice has it backwards. In ethics, the true route begins with practice,

---

* "Thinking (*dianoia*) itself moves nothing, but only thinking for the sake of something and practical (*praktike*); for this is the governing source (*arche*) also of productive activity (*poietike*). . . . Now, regarding the thing done (*to prakton*) acting-well is the end, and desire (or appetite; *orexis*) is for this. Therefore, *choice* (*proairesis*)—[the source of action]—is either appetitive intellect (*orektikos nous*) or thoughtful appetite (*orexis dianoetike*), and a human being (*anthropos*) is such a principle (or source; *arche*)." (*Nicomachean Ethics*, 1139a36–b7)

with deeds and doers, and moves only secondarily to reflection on practice. Indeed, even the propensity to *care* about moral matters requires a certain *moral disposition,* acquired in practice, before the age of reflection arrives. As Aristotle points out, he who has "the that" can easily get "the why." Moreover, because this sort of philosophical reflection mirrors genuine conduct, ethics would not become wholly or purely abstract, would never reach to what we call ethical theory, because it would retain its connection with the concreteness and complexities of the moral life and the moral agent. This more or less neglected approach to ethics deserves our attention, especially if we mean to make a practical moral difference. We must consider that the real action in practicing ethics will begin when we again see ethics as practice, as the putting-to-work of character and custom, in conduct that both creates and manifests the human agent, thoughtfully-at-work negotiating the many challenges of the human condition.

### Habits of Affection and Behavior: Toward a Different Practice of Ethics

The contrast I am suggesting between the two meanings of practicing ethics—ethics as theory with application; ethics as practice with reflection—parallels the contrast between two forms of our moral life described by Michael Oakeshott in a marvelous essay, "The Tower of Babel."[1] Oakeshott contrasts the moral life as a habit of affection and behavior and the moral life as the self-conscious and reflective application of a moral criterion, and he tries to show the disadvantages we suffer because of our culture's growing emphasis on the latter at the expense of the former. As the second is familiar and in tune with our present preferences, let me speak only about the first, with Oakeshott's help. In the moral life understood through habits of affection and conduct,

> [t]he current situations of moral life are met, not by consciously applying to ourselves a rule of behaviour, nor by conduct recognized as the expression of a moral ideal, but by acting in accordance with a certain habit of behaviour. The moral life in this form does not spring from the consciousness of possible

alternative ways of behaving and a choice, determined by an opinion, a rule or an ideal, from among these alternatives; conduct is as nearly as possible without reflection. And consequently, most of the current situations of life do not appear as occasions calling for judgment, or as problems requiring solutions; there is no weighing up of alternatives or reflection on consequences, no uncertainty, no battle of scruples. There is, on the occasion, nothing more than the unreflective following of a tradition of conduct in which we have been brought up.... I am describing the form which moral action takes (because it can take no other) in all the emergencies of life when time and opportunity for reflection are lacking, and I am supposing that what is true of the emergencies of life is true of most of the occasions when human conduct is free from natural necessity.[2]

Moral life here flows from character—ingrained, concrete, steady, like a second nature. And although the conduct it yields is not the product of reasoning, it is nonetheless (or, perhaps, therefore) utterly reasonable and fitting. Though not rationalist, it makes immediate sense.

How is this form of moral life acquired? Not by philosophizing, not by doing "values clarification" or laying out ethical theory, not by applying theory to practice, but from education of a certain sort:

We acquire habits of conduct, not by constructing a way of living upon rules or precepts learned by heart and subsequently practised, but *by living with people who habitually behave in a certain manner:* we acquire habits of conduct in the same way as we acquire our native language. There is no point in a child's life at which he can be said to begin to learn the language which is habitually spoken in his hearing; and there is no point in his life at which he can be said to begin to learn habits of behaviour from the people constantly about him. No doubt, in both cases, what is learnt (or some of it) can be formulated in rules and precepts; but in neither case do we, in this kind of education, learn by learning rules and precepts.... [I]f we have acquired a knowledge of the rules, this sort of command of language and behaviour is impossible until we have forgotten them as rules and are *no longer tempted to turn speech and action into the applications of rules to a situation.* Further, the education by means of which we acquire habits of affection and behaviour is not only coeval with conscious life, but it is carried on, in practice and observation, without pause in every moment of our waking life, and perhaps even in our dreams; what is begun as imitation continues as selective conformity to a rich variety of customary behaviour. This sort of education is not compulsory; it is inevitable.... [I]t is the sort of education which gives the power to act appropriately and without hesitation, doubt or difficulty, but which does not give the ability to explain our actions in abstract terms, or defend them as emanations of moral principles.... And a man may be said to have acquired most thoroughly what this kind of moral education can teach him *when his moral dispositions are inseverably connected with his amour-propre,* when the spring of his conduct is not an attachment to an ideal or a felt duty to obey a rule, but his self-esteem, and when to act wrongly is felt as diminution of his self-esteem.[3]

Habitual practice informs its source: heart-and-mind are together dyed fast by repeated immersions in the practice of daily living.

Oakeshott's point about *amour-propre* and self-esteem is crucial: practicing ethics in this full sense is nothing less than full self-expression, the manifestation of who one is at one's core. It points to the need for institutions that cultivate self-esteem and, more to the point, give *moral content* to our self-esteem, that make us believe that acting rightly is not just the other fellow's good but our own true flourishing. Early family life, schools, churches and synagogues, colleges, voluntary associations and professional societies all have roles to play in such moral education, less by the elaboration of doctrine, more by the encouragement and reward of seemly and decent conduct and sensibilities. And while speech and philosophy have a role to play here, we should not exaggerate their power.

At the end of his *Nicomachean Ethics,* a deeply reflective work on the active life which indeed tries to explain "the why" to those well-brought-up readers who already have "the that," Aristotle shows why ethics is impotent without politics—without careful attention to law and custom and the ordering of civic life. He makes his turn toward law and politics by remarking on the weakness of speech, including philosophical speech, presumably including also his own.

If speeches [or arguments or discourses on ethics] were sufficient to make men decent, "large fees and many" justly "would
they win" (according to Theognis), and to provide such
[speeches] would be all that is needed. But it appears that
speeches have influence to encourage and stimulate the liberal
youth, and given an inborn good character and a true love of
the noble, they might make him capable of being possessed by
virtue, but they are incapable of stimulating the many toward
nobility. For they are not natured to be obedient to reverence
[or awe-ful shame; *aidos*] but to fear, and to abstain from evil
not because of its baseness but on account of the penalties.
(1179b4–13)

Speeches and arguments are at best influential only with those
already well disposed toward the noble or the just; for the many,
fear of penalty takes the place of reverence or awe-shame. But in
both cases, the crucial matter for moral education is the ruling passion of people's souls. Ethics must concern itself especially with how
these passions are formed and addressed.

Where is it that human beings are encouraged in reverence or
awe? Where is it that human beings are stretched toward a vision
of something better or higher or finer? Could it be that something
like piety—familial, civil, religious—is a crucial ingredient in the
most responsive moral souls? And what of the others? Do we not
need the development of laws and customs with proper sanctions—
*logoi* with teeth—to help guide those not amenable to persuasion?

These reflections point to the central need for attention to institutions—familial, religious, political. Indeed, one of the most astonishing things to me in the entire field of bioethics is how
unpsychological and, especially, unpolitical are its reflections. And
yet the character of our regime, the things we honor and reward,
deplore and punish, deeply influence—albeit not always in obvious
ways—the sorts of moral agents we become as individuals. Ethics
will never be efficacious in action until we start attending to these
matters.

## Where's the Action for Tomorrow?

If my analysis is correct, even partly correct, it points to new are-
nas for ethical action and new challenges of leadership for the field
of bioethics. To be sure, these new challenges will also require careful thought, but thought of a somewhat different kind—let us say
"strategic" rather than "theoretic." We need to think less about *doctrine* and *principles* and the rules to govern behavior, more about
*education* and *institutions*—and what sort of people we produce.
We need to think about how to encourage and enhance the formation of certain sentiments and attitudes. If there is a greater need for
respect, reverence and gravity, or for trust, sympathy and tolerance,
we need to think about what produces these things and what undermines them. We need to think about how to strengthen and defend
those mediating structures and institutions which cultivate the habits
of moral affections and conduct—especially family, the Scouts, religious institutions, civic and public-service associations, and the like.
It may turn out, for instance, that changes in divorce law or child-
care practices are ethically far more deserving of our attention than
arguments about the status of the *in vitro* embryo or the rights of
its biological progenitors. It may turn out that designing programs
of compensated national service for our high school graduates
deserves as much of our ethical attention as the ethics of various
techniques of behavior modification. Such examples could be multiplied at will.

What I am talking about is, of course, nothing less than concern for the moral health of our entire community. We should therefore have no illusions about how much any one organization can
contribute, or indeed, about how well the best national effort of the
best hearts and minds can succeed. Indeed, I now appreciate a remark
made thirty years ago by my cousin when I told him why I was entering the field of medical ethics: "You think you can do something
about *this?* This is work for Mashiyach [the Messiah]."

Yet if we look concretely into our own front yard—medical
ethics—there is, it seems to me, much constructive inquiry and action
to be taken. We can give special attention to institutions and customs that help shape medical practice and, especially, that shape the

attitudes, sensibilities and habits of medical practitioners as moral agents. We could tackle the question of how prospective physicians, nurses, biomedical scientists and hospital administrators are recruited and educated. We could seek to find appropriate studies to deepen their understanding of the meaning of our humanity. Is it from works of dry reason or from works of reasonable feeling—that is, is it from philosophy professors John Rawls and Richard Rorty or from the Bible and Tolstoy—that we best cultivate moral sentiments and sensibilities? What sort and manner of humanistic learning truly humanizes? We could also concern ourselves with questions like the following: What sorts of performances and outlooks are and should be esteemed in the medical admissions process? What is praised and blamed, honored and held shameful, in medical training and medical practice? How can one bring new physicians into more apprentice-like relations with master physicians? What are the criteria for licensure and board certification, and, hence, what sorts of character do they encourage? What is the substructure of hospitals and medical associations, and how do they influence and sanction conduct, sentiments, attitudes? What sort of examples form our culture's perception of medicine? Does it matter whether it comes mainly from Dr. Killdare or from General Hospital? What can be done, institutionally, to foster greater trust and responsiveness between physicians and patients? (A comparable set of questions could be raised about the moral and humanistic education of biomedical scientists and biotechnologists.)

These questions about institutions and their effects on character are extremely complicated, and lack the neatness of abstract theory. Yet if we mean to do something about action, if we mean to practice ethics in a way that will yield a more ethical medical practice, we must devote at least some of our energies to these matters. We will not even know the possibilities here until we try, and try we must.

## *Renewing Moral Capital, Seeking Moral Wisdom*

For most of this analysis, I have been criticizing the rationalist talk of academic ethicists in the name of genuine moral action, performed by countless people in everyday life. Yet the field of bioethics also deserves criticism in the domain of thought, where its penchant for problem solving and regulation has deflected it from the profound matters that gave rise to the field thirty years ago. Today, the public, taking its bearings from lived experience, rather than the bioethics profession, drunk on abstract theory, has a better idea of why the biological revolution and biotechnology are humanly important and deserving of the most concerned attention.

Indeed, few issues over the past three decades have captured public attention like those of bioethics. Yet the reason for their prominence, I submit, has little to do with the rationalist notions and approaches promulgated by most practicing bioethicists. On the contrary, the public concern with bioethics is at once more immediate and more profound. It begins with the concrete existential questions surrounding birth and death, sickness and health, suffering and flourishing. But it knowingly reaches down—even if only tacitly—to the central concerns of human life: identity and individuality, freedom and finitude, embodiment and selfhood, sexuality and procreation, and the deeply mysterious longings of the human soul. Yet lacking a master cultural and moral narrative that can guide us through the minefields of the biotechnological revolution, we turn to the "experts" in bioethics in the hope of gaining clarity about what this all means and wisdom about what we must do to keep human life human. So far, the field of bioethics has let us down.

If the field of bioethics is to respond properly to the deepest challenges raised by biomedical science and technology, it will have to draw on moral capital of a different, less academic sort. And it will have to philosophize in a more venerable mode, reviving a more natural way of thinking feelingly and a more direct engagement with the first of the philosophical questions, made famous by Socrates, the question of "How to Live." It will have to live up to the original meaning and purpose of philosophy, the seeking of moral wisdom, now urgently needed more than ever if we are to live well in the face of the new challenges of biotechnology.

Our rationalistic theoretical activities, for all their clarity, are by their very abstractness and their preoccupation with problem solving, incapable of contributing to the increase or renewal of the needed moral capital or the passionate pursuit of wisdom. To the contrary, our activities are in danger of undermining them: sometimes explicitly by, say, the condescension shown by bioethicists for habitual practice, moral sentiment, or religious insights, more often by sheer indifference or neglect. We may, in the end, be incapable of stemming the rationalist prejudice, so prevalent in our age, or of revitalizing those institutions that lay the moral foundations of private and public life. But we would be at fault for not seeing the need to do so.

The field of bioethics faces a not atypical problem of perpetuation: how to provide for the kinds of people and moral concerns that got it started. People like physician Henry Beecher, theologian Paul Ramsey, philosopher Hans Jonas, physician Andre Hellegers, biologist and educator Robert Morison, ethicist and writer Dan Callahan, and psychoanalyst Will Gaylin were, to repeat, not brought up on bioethics or moral theory, and no academic training accounts for their vision, courage and moral passion. They helped institutionalize a world of ethical discourse that might give the impression that *their* moral beginnings are no longer necessary. Nothing could be further from the truth. We must return to what animated the enterprise: the fears, the hopes, the distastes, the moral concern and, above all, the recognition that beneath the distinctive issues of bioethics lie the deepest matters of our humanity. We must constantly remind ourselves of what it is that we wish humanly to defend and preserve, always keeping in view the defining and worthy features of human life. Nothing less deserves to be called "bioethics," the ethics of human life as humanly lived.

# ✻ Ethical Challenges
# from Biotechnology

# ❖ Life and Lineage: Genetics and the Beginning of Life

# CHAPTER THREE

# The Meaning of Life—
# in the Laboratory

*People will not look forward to posterity who never look backward to
their ancestors. —Edmund Burke*

*What's a nice embryo like you doing in a place like this? —Traditional*

The readers of Aldous Huxley's novel, like the inhabitants of the society it depicts, enter into the Brave New World through "a squat gray building . . . the Central London Hatchery and Conditioning Centre," beginning, in fact, in the Fertilizing Room. There, three hundred fertilizers sit bent over their instruments, inspecting eggs, immersing them "in warm bouillon containing free-swimming spermatozoa," and incubating the successfully fertilized eggs until they are ripe for bottling (or Bokanovskification). Here, most emphatically, life begins with fertilization—in the laboratory. Life in the laboratory is the gateway to the Brave New World.

We stand today fully on the threshold of that gateway. How far and how fast we should continue to travel through this entrance is not a matter of chance or necessity but rather a matter of human decision—*our* human decision. Indeed, it seems to be reserved to the people of this country and this century, by our conduct and example, to decide also this important question.

Should we allow or encourage the initiation and growth of human life in the laboratory? This question, in one form or another, has been an issue for public policy since the mid-1970s, even before the birth of the first test-tube baby in the summer of 1978. Back in 1975, after prolonged deliberations, the National Commission for the Protection of Human Subjects of Biomedical and Behavioral

Research issued its report and recommendations for research on the human fetus. The Secretary of Health, Education and Welfare (HEW) then published regulations regarding research, development and related activities involving fetuses, pregnant women and *in vitro* fertilization. These provided that no federal monies should be used for *in vitro* fertilization of human eggs until a special Ethics Advisory Board reviewed the ethical issues and offered advice about whether government should support any such proposed research. Perhaps for the first time in the modern era of biomedical research, public deliberation and debate about ethical matters led to an effective moratorium on federal support for experimentation.

A few years later, the whole matter once again became the subject of intense policy debate when an Ethics Advisory Board was established to consider whether the United States government should finance research on human life in the laboratory. The question had been placed on the policy table by a research proposal submitted to the National Institute of Child Health and Human Development by Dr. Pierre Soupart of Vanderbilt University. Dr. Soupart requested $465,000 for a study to define in part the genetic risk involved in obtaining early human embryos by tissue culture methods. He proposed to fertilize about 450 human ova, obtained from donors undergoing gynecological surgery (that is, not from women whom the research could be expected to help), with donor sperm, to observe their development for five to six days, and to examine them microscopically for chromosomal and other abnormalities before discarding them. In addition, he planned to study whether such laboratory-grown embryos could be frozen and stored without introducing abnormalities, for it was thought that temporary cold storage of human embryos might improve the success rate in the subsequent embryo transfer procedure used to produce a child. Though Dr. Soupart did not then propose to perform embryo transfers for women seeking to become pregnant, his research was intended to serve that goal: he hoped to reassure us that baby-making with the help of *in vitro* fertilization was safe, and he sought to perfect the techniques of laboratory growth of human embryos introduced by Drs. Robert Edwards and Patrick Steptoe in England.

Dr. Soupart's application was approved for funding by the National Institutes of Health (NIH) in October 1977, but because of the administrative regulations, it could not be funded without review by an Ethics Advisory Board. The HEW secretary at the time, Joseph Califano, convened such a board and charged it not only with a decision on the Soupart proposal, but with an inquiry into all the scientific, ethical and legal issues involved, urging it "to provide recommendations on broad principles to guide the Department in future decision-making." After six months of public hearings all over the United States and another six months of private deliberation, the board issued its report in 1979, recommending that research funding be permitted for some *in vitro* experimentation—including the sort proposed by Dr. Soupart. But until very recently, no secretary of health and human services has been willing to act on that recommendation. In fact, Dr. Soupart died in 1981 without having received a clear answer from the government.

There the matter stood until 1994. In the previous year, Congress and President Clinton had for the first time given NIH the authority to support research on human embryos. In response, NIH established the Human Embryo Research Panel to assess the moral and ethical issues raised by this research and to develop recommendations and guidelines for the agency's review. In September 1994 the panel released its report, recommending that some areas of human embryo research be acceptable for federal funding, including research on embryos *created expressly for the purposes of research,* under certain limited conditions. Two months later, the Advisory Committee to the Director of NIH unanimously accepted the panel's report. However, President Clinton directed NIH *not* to allocate resources to "support the creation of human embryos for research purposes," though his directive said nothing about research involving so-called "spare" embryos remaining from clinical *in vitro* fertilization procedures performed to help infertile couples become parents. While NIH was in the process of developing guidelines to support research using those "spare" embryos, Congress stopped the enterprise dead in its tracks by enacting an amendment to the omnibus appropriations bills that prohibited NIH from using federal funds for *any* and *all* research on human embryos. Similar congressional prohibitions have been enacted in every year since then. Meanwhile, private-sector research using human embryos was heating up, yielding some remarkable discoveries that would soon reignite the controversy about federal funding for human embryo research.

In November 1998, Dr. James Thomson of the University of Wisconsin and Dr. John Gearhart of Johns Hopkins University announced the isolation of human embryonic stem cells, so-called pluripotent cells extracted from human embryos that are capable of being turned into any of the tissues of the body. As a result of this capacity, these cells are widely believed to hold great promise for regenerative medicine—the replacement of damaged tissues responsible for many horrible genetic or chronic diseases or disabilities. With this discovery, privately funded research on human embryos went into high gear, and federally funded researchers looked for ways to circumvent the legislative prohibition. By a clever interpretation of the law that went against its spirit but not its letter, NIH attorneys ruled that the prohibiting law actually permitted federal funding of research on the embryonic stem cell *lines,* provided that the researchers were not themselves responsible for the acts of embryo destruction needed to produce them. After a study by the National Bioethics Advisory Commission supported such research, and after the NIH developed guidelines for it, President Clinton authorized such funding in 2000.

Then, a newly elected President Bush announced early in 2001 that he would review the matter before permitting implementation of the NIH plan. During the following six months of deliberation, President Bush consulted widely with persons holding every imaginable viewpoint on the subject, as he sought to find a solution to his moral dilemma: how to allow federally funded scientists an opportunity to find out whether embryonic stem cells could indeed deliver on their therapeutic promise, while at the same time upholding his strong belief that nascent life should not be destroyed in the process. In August 2001, he announced his solution. The federal government would agree to fund embryonic stem cell research only on already existing stem cell lines, but there would be no cooperation in, and no abetting of, any further destruction of human embryos. That is where things stand as this book goes to press, though it is almost certain that we have not heard the end of the matter. The existing stem cell lines might age and wither; newly derived cell lines may show more promise than the existing ones; and other important uses for human embryos in research and treatment will no doubt be discovered. It is almost as certain as death and taxes that we shall experience enormous pressures to grow more and more life in the laboratory. It is thus extremely important that we think about the meaning of doing so and assess the moral arguments for and against.

## *The Meaning of the Question*

How should one think about such ethical matters, here and in general? There are many possible ways, and it is not altogether clear which way is best. For some people, ethical issues are immediately matters of right and wrong, of purity and sin, of good and evil. For others, the critical terms are benefits and harms, promises and risks, gains and costs. Some will focus on so-called rights of individuals or groups (for example, a right to life or childbirth); still others will emphasize supposed goods for society and its members, such as the advancement of knowledge and the prevention and cure of disease. My own orientation here is somewhat different. I wish to suggest that before deciding what to do, one should try to understand the implications of doing or not doing. The first task, it seems to me, is not to ask "moral or immoral?" or "right or wrong?" but to try to understand fully the meaning and significance of the proposed actions.

This concern with significance leads me to take a broad view of the matter. For we are concerned here not only with some limited research project of the sort proposed by Dr. Soupart, and the narrow issues of safety and informed consent it immediately raises; we are concerned also with a whole range of implications, including many that are tied to foreseeable consequences of this research and its predictable extensions—and touching even our common conception of our own humanity. As most of us are at least tacitly aware, more is at stake than in ordinary biomedical research or in experimenting with human subjects at risk of bodily harm. At stake is the *idea* of the *humanness* of our human life and the meaning of our embodiment, our sexual being, and our relation to ancestors and descendants. In thinking about necessarily particular and immediate decisions, we must be mindful of the larger picture and must avoid the great danger of trivializing the matter for the sake of rendering it manageable.

## *The Status of Extracorporeal Life*

The meaning of "life in the laboratory" turns in part on the nature and meaning of the human embryo, isolated in the laboratory and separate from the confines of a woman's body. What is the status of a fertilized human egg (that is, a human zygote) and the embryo that develops from it? How are we to regard its being? How are we to regard it morally (that is, how are we to behave toward it)? These are, alas, all too familiar questions. At least analogous, if not identical, questions are central to the abortion controversy and are also crucial in considering whether and what sort of experimentation is properly conducted on living but aborted fetuses. Would that it were possible to say that the matter is simple and obvious, and that it has been resolved to everyone's satisfaction!

But the controversy about the morality of abortion continues to rage and divide our nation. Moreover, many who favor or at least do not oppose abortion do so despite the fact that they regard the pre-viable fetus as a living human organism, even if less worthy of protection than a woman's desire not to give it birth. Almost everyone senses the importance of this matter for the decision about laboratory culture of and experimentation with human embryos. Thus, we are obliged to take up the question of the status of the embryo in our search for the outlines of some common ground on which many of us can stand. To the best of my knowledge, the discussion that follows is not informed by any particular sectarian or religious teaching, though it may perhaps reveal that I am a person not devoid of reverence and the capacity for awe and wonder, said by some to be the core of the religious sentiment.

I begin by noting that the circumstances of laboratory-grown blastocysts (that is, three-to-six-day-old embryos, containing from 100 to 200 cells) and embryos are not identical with those of the analogous cases of living fetuses facing abortion or living aborted fetuses used in research. First, the fetuses whose fates are at issue in abortion are unwanted, usually the result of "accidental" conception. The lab-grown embryos are wanted and deliberately created, despite certain knowledge that many of them will be destroyed or discarded. Moreover, the fate of these embryos is not in conflict with the wishes, interests or alleged rights of the pregnant women. Second, though the federal guidelines governing fetal research permit studies conducted on the not-at-all viable aborted fetus, such research merely takes advantage of available "products" of abortions not themselves undertaken for the sake of the research. No one has proposed and no one would sanction the deliberate production of live fetuses to be aborted for the sake of research—even very beneficial research.* In contrast, we are here considering the deliberate production of embryos for the express purpose of experimentation.

The cases may also differ in other ways. Given the present state of the art, the largest embryo under discussion is the blastocyst, a spherical, relatively undifferentiated mass of cells, barely visible to the naked eye. In appearance, it does not look human; indeed, only the most careful scrutiny by the most experienced scientist might distinguish it from similar blastocysts of other mammals. If the human zygote and blastocyst are more like the animal zygote and blastocyst than like the twelve-week-old human fetus (which already has a humanoid appearance, differentiated organs and electrical activity of the brain), then there will be a much-diminished ethical dilemma regarding their deliberate creation and experimental use. Needless to say, there are articulate and passionate defenders of all points of view. Let us try, however, to consider the matter afresh.

First of all, the zygote and early embryonic stages are clearly alive. They metabolize, respire and respond to changes in the environment; they grow and divide. Second, though not yet organized into distinctive parts or organs, the blastocyst is an organic whole, self-developing, genetically unique and distinct from the egg and sperm whose union marked the beginning of its career as a discrete, unfolding being. While the egg and sperm are alive as cells, something new and alive *in a different sense* comes into being with fertilization. The truth of this is unaffected by the fact that fertilization takes time and is not an instantaneous event. For after fertilization is *complete,* there exists a new individual, with its unique genetic

---

*Though perhaps a justifiable exception would be a universal plague that fatally attacked all fetuses *in utero.* To find a cure for the end of the species may entail deliberately "producing" (and aborting) live fetuses for research.

identity, fully potent for the self-initiated development into a mature human being, if circumstances are cooperative. Though there is some sense in which the lives of egg and sperm are continuous with the life of the new organism (or, in human terms, that the parents live on in the child-to-be), in the decisive sense there is a discontinuity, a new beginning, with fertilization. *After* fertilization, there is continuity of subsequent development, even if the locus of the new living being alters with implantation (or birth). Any honest biologist must be impressed by these facts, and must be inclined, at least on first glance, to the view that a human life begins at fertilization.\* Even Dr. Robert Edwards had apparently stumbled over this truth, perhaps inadvertently, in his remark about Louise Brown, his first successful test-tube baby: "The last time I saw *her, she* was just eight cells in a test-tube. *She* was beautiful *then,* and she's still beautiful *now!*"

Granting that a human life begins at fertilization and develops via a continuous process thereafter, surely—one might say—the blastocyst itself can hardly be considered a human being. I myself would agree that a blastocyst is not, in a *full* sense, a human being— or what the current fashion calls, rather arbitrarily and without clear definition, a person. It does not look like a human being nor can it do very much of what human beings do. Yet, at the same time, I must acknowledge that the human blastocyst is (1) human in origin and (2) *potentially* a mature human being, if all goes well. This, too, is beyond dispute; indeed, it is precisely because of its peculiarly human potentialities that people propose to study *it* rather than the embryos of other mammals. The human blastocyst, even the human blastocyst *in vitro,* is not humanly nothing; it possesses a power to become what everyone will agree is a human being. One could even go further: the *in vitro* blastocyst is exactly what a human being is at that stage of human development. Only its extracorporeal location is different.

---

\*The truth of this is not decisively affected by the fact that the early embryo may soon divide and give rise to identical twins or by the fact that scientists may disaggregate and reassemble the cells of the early embryos, even mixing in cells from different embryos in the reaggregation. These unusual and artificial cases do not affect the natural norm, or the truth that a human life begins with fertilization—and does so always, if nothing abnormal occurs.

Because of the embryo's special location, it may be objected that the blastocyst *in vitro* has today no such power, because there is presently no *in vitro* way to bring the blastocyst to that much later fetal stage in which it might survive on its own. There are no published reports of the culture of human embryos past the blastocyst stage (though this has been reported for mice). The *in vitro* blastocyst, like the twelve-week-old aborted fetus, is *in this sense* not viable (in other words, it is at a stage of maturation before the stage of possible independent existence). But if, among the not-viable embryos, we distinguish between the *pre*-viable and the *not-at-all* viable—on the basis that the former, though not yet viable, is capable of becoming or being made viable—we note a crucial difference between the blastocyst and the twelve-week-old abortus. Unlike an aborted fetus, the blastocyst is possibly salvageable, and hence potentially viable, *if it is transferred to a woman for implantation*. It is not strictly true that the *in vitro* blastocyst is *necessarily* not viable. Until proven otherwise, by embryo transfer and attempted implantation, we are right to consider the human blastocyst *in vitro* as potentially a human being and, in this respect, not fundamentally different from a blastocyst *in utero*. To put the matter more forcefully, the blastocyst *in vitro* is more viable, in the sense of more salvageable, than aborted fetuses at most later stages up to, say, twenty weeks.

This is not to assert that such a blastocyst is therefore endowed with a "right to life," that failure to implant it is negligent homicide, or that experimental touchings of such blastocysts constitute assault and battery. (I myself tend to reject such claims, and indeed think that the ethical questions are not best posed in terms of rights.) But the blastocyst is not nothing; it is *at least* potential humanity, and as such it elicits, or ought to elicit, our feelings of awe and respect. In the blastocyst, even in the zygote, we face a mysterious and awesome power, a power governed by an immanent plan that may produce an indisputably and fully human being. It deserves our respect not because it has rights or claims or sentience (which it does not have at this stage), but because of what it is, now and prospectively.

Let us test this provisional conclusion by considering intuitively our response to two possible fates of such zygotes, blastocysts and early embryos. First, should such an embryo die, will we be inclined to mourn its passing? When a woman we know miscarries, we are sad—largely for *her* loss and disappointment, but perhaps also at the premature death of a life that might have been. But we do not mourn the departed fetus, nor do we seek ritually to dispose of the remains. In this respect, we do not treat even the fetus as fully one of us.

On the other hand, we would, I suppose, recoil even from the thought, let alone the practice—I apologize for forcing it upon the reader—of eating such embryos, should someone discover that they would constitute a great delicacy, a "human caviar." The human blastocyst would be protected by our taboo against cannibalism, which insists on the humanness of human flesh and does not permit us to treat even the flesh of the dead as if it were mere meat. *The human embryo is not mere meat; it is not just stuff; it is not a "thing."** Because of its origin and because of its capacity, it commands a higher respect.

How much more respect? As much as for a fully developed human being? My own inclination is to say probably not, but who can be certain? Indeed, there might be prudential and reasonable grounds for an affirmative answer, partly because the presumption of ignorance ought to err in the direction of never underestimating the basis for respect of human life (not least, for our own self-respect), partly because so many people feel very strongly that even the blastocyst is protectably human. As a first approximation, I would analogize the early embryo *in vitro* to the early embryo *in utero* (because both are potentially viable and human). On this ground alone, the most sensible policy is to *treat the early embryo as a pre-viable fetus, with constraints imposed on early embryo research at least as great as those on fetal research.*

---

*Some people have suggested that the embryo be regarded in the same manner as a vital organ, salvaged from a newly dead corpse, usable for transplantation or research, and that its donation by egg and sperm donors be governed by the Uniform Anatomical Gift Act, which legitimates premortem consent for organ donation upon death. But though this acknowledges that embryos are not "things," it is a mistake to treat embryos as mere organs, thereby overlooking that they are early stages of a complete, whole human being. The Uniform Anatomical Gift Act does not apply to, nor should it be stretched to cover, donation of gonads, gametes (male sperm or female eggs) or—especially—zygotes and embryos.

To some this may seem excessively scrupulous. They will point to the absence of a distinctive humanoid appearance or the absence of sentience. To be sure, we would feel more restraint in invasive procedures conducted on a five-month-old or even a twelve-week-old living fetus than on a blastocyst. But this added restraint on inflicting suffering on a look-alike, feeling creature in no way denies the propriety of a prior restraint, grounded in respect for individuated, living, potential humanity. Before I would be persuaded to treat early embryos differently from later ones, I would insist on the establishment of a reasonably clear, naturally grounded boundary that would separate "early" and "late," and on the provision of a basis for respecting the "early" less than the "late." This burden must be accepted by proponents of experimentation with human embryos *in vitro* if a decision to permit the creation of embryos for such experimentation is to be treated as ethically responsible.

## The Treatment of Extracorporeal Embryos

Where does the above analysis lead in thinking about treatment of human embryos in the laboratory? I indicate, very briefly, the lines toward a possible policy, though that is not my major intent.

The *in vitro* fertilized embryo has four possible fates: (1) implantation, in the hope of producing from it a child; (2) death, by active killing or disaggregation, or by a "natural" demise; (3) use in manipulative experimentation—embryological, genetic, extraction of stem cells, etc.; and (4) use in attempts at perpetuation *in vitro* beyond the blastocyst stage, ultimately, perhaps, to viability. Let us consider each in turn.

On the strength of my analysis of the status of the embryo and the respect due it, no objection would be raised to implantation. *in vitro* fertilization and embryo transfer to treat infertility—as in the case of Mr. and Mrs. Brown, now repeated tens of thousands of times—is perfectly compatible with a respect and reverence for human life, including potential human life. Moreover, no disrespect is intended or practiced by the mere fact that several eggs are removed to increase the chance of success. Were it possible to guarantee successful fertilization and normal growth with a single egg, no more would need to be obtained. Assuming nothing further is done with the unimplanted embryos, there is nothing disrespectful going on. The demise of the unimplanted embryos would be analogous to the loss of numerous embryos wasted in the normal *in vivo* attempts to generate a child. It is estimated that over 50 percent of eggs successfully fertilized during unprotected sexual intercourse fail to implant, or do not remain implanted, in the uterine wall, and are shed soon thereafter, before a diagnosis of pregnancy could be made. Any couple attempting to conceive a child tacitly accepts the sad fact of such embryonic wastage as the perfectly tolerable price to be paid for the birth of a (usually) healthy child. Current procedures to initiate pregnancy with laboratory fertilization thus differ from the natural process in that what would normally be spread over four or five months *in vivo* is compressed into a single effort, using all at once a four or five months' supply of eggs.*

Parenthetically, we should note that the natural occurrence of embryo and fetal loss and wastage does not necessarily or automatically justify all deliberate, humanly caused destruction of fetal life. For example, the natural loss of embryos in early pregnancy cannot in itself be a warrant for deliberately aborting them or for invasively experimenting on them *in vitro*, any more than stillbirths could be a justification for newborn infanticide. There are many things that happen naturally that we ought not do deliberately. It is curious how the same people who deny the relevance of nature as a guide for evaluating human interventions into human generation, and who deny that the term "unnatural" carries any ethical weight, will themselves appeal to "nature's way" when it suits their

---

*The problem of surplus embryos may someday be avoidable, for purely technical reasons. Some researchers believe that uterine receptivity to the transferred embryo might be reduced during the menstrual cycle in which the ova are obtained because of the effects of the hormones given to induce superovulation. They propose that the harvested eggs be frozen and then defrosted one at a time each month for fertilization, culture and transfer, until pregnancy is achieved. By refusing to fertilize all the eggs at once—not placing all one's eggs in one uterine cycle—there would not be surplus embryos, but only surplus eggs. This change in procedure would make the demise of unimplanted embryos exactly analogous to the "natural" embryonic loss in ordinary reproduction. Unfortunately, a method of freezing and thawing eggs without destroying them has yet to be found.

purposes.* Still, in this present matter, the closeness to natural pro-creation—the goal is the same, the embryonic loss is unavoidable and not desired, and the amount of loss is similar—leads me to believe that we do no more intentional or unjustified harm in one case than in the other and we practice no disrespect.

But must we allow the unimplanted *in vitro* embryos to die? Why should they not be either transferred for adoption into another infertile woman, or else used for investigative purposes, to seek new knowledge, say, about gene action in health or disease, or to extract stem cells to be developed for possible use in regenerative medicine? The first option raises questions about lineage and the nature of par-enthood to which I will return. But even on first glance, it would seem likely to raise a large objection from the original couple who were seeking a child of their own and not the dissemination of their biological children for prenatal adoption.

But what about experimentation on such blastocysts and early embryos? Is that compatible with the respect they deserve? This is the hard question. On balance, I would think not. Invasive and manipulative experiments involving such embryos very likely pre-sume that they are things or mere stuff and deny the fact of their possible viability. Certain observational and noninvasive experi-ments might be different. But on the whole, I would think that the respect for human embryos for which I have argued—not, I repeat, their "right to life"—would lead one to oppose most potentially interesting and useful experimentation. This is a dilemma, and one which cannot be ducked or defined away. Either we accept certain great restrictions on the permissible uses of human embryos or we deliberately decide to override—though I hope not deny—the respect due to the embryos.

I am aware that I have pointed toward a seemingly paradox-ical conclusion about the treatment of the unimplanted embryos:

---

*The literature on intervention in reproduction is both confused and confusing on the crucial matter of the meanings of "nature" or "the natural," and their significance for the ethical issues. It may be as much a mistake to claim that the natural has no moral force as to suggest that the natural way is best, because natural. Though shallow and slippery thought about nature, and its relation to "good," is a likely source of these confusions, the nature of nature may itself be elusive, making it difficult for even careful thought to capture what is natural.

Leave them alone, and do not create embryos for experimentation only. To let them die naturally would be the most respectful course, grounded on a reverence, generically, for their potential humanity, and a respect, individually, for their being the seed and offspring of a particular couple, who were themselves seeking only to have a child of their own. An analysis that stressed a right to life, rather than respect, would, of course, lead to different conclusions. Only an analysis of the embryo's status that denies both its so-called rights and its worthiness of all respect would have no trouble sanctioning its use in investigative research, donation to other couples, stem cell extraction, commercial transactions and other such activities.

　　I have to this point ignored the fourth potential fate of life in the laboratory: perpetuation in the bottle beyond the blastocyst state, perhaps ultimately to viability. As a practical matter, this repugnant Huxleyan prospect probably need not concern us much for the time being. But as a thought experiment, it permits us to test further our intuitions about the meaning of life in the laboratory and to discover thereby the limitations of the previous analysis. For these unimplanted, cultivated embryos raise even more profound difficulties. Bad as it may now be to discard or experiment upon them in these primordial stages, it would be far worse to perpetuate them to later stages in their laboratory existence—especially when the technology arrives that can bring them to viability *in vitro*. For how long and up to what stage of development will they be considered fit material for experimentation? When ought they to be released from the machinery and admitted into the human fraternity, or, at least, into the premature nursery? The need for a respectable boundary defining protectable human life cannot be overstated. The current boundaries, gerrymandered for the sake of abortion—namely, birth or viability—may now satisfy both women's liberation and the United States Supreme Court and may someday satisfy even a future pope, but they will not survive the coming of more sophisticated technologies for growing life in the laboratory.*

---

*In *Roe v. Wade*, the Supreme Court ruled that state action regarding abortion was unconstitutional in the first trimester of pregnancy, permissible after the first trimester in order to promote the health of the "mother," and permissible in order to protect "potential life" only at viability (about 24 weeks), prior to which time the state's interest in fetal life was deemed not "compelling." This rather careless and arbitrary placement of boundaries is already something of an embarrassment, thanks to

But what if perpetuation in the laboratory were to be sought not for the sake of experimentation but in order to produce a healthy living child—say, one with all the benefits of a scientifically based gestational nourishment and care? Would such treatment of a laboratory-grown embryo be compatible with the respect it is owed? If we consider only what is owed to its vitality and potential humanity *as an individuated human being,* then the laboratory growth of an embryo into a viable full-term baby (that is, ectogenesis) would be perfectly compatible with the requisite respect. (Indeed, for these reasons one would guess that the right-to-life people, who object even to the destruction of blastocysts, would find infinitely preferable any form of their preservation and perpetuation to term, in the bottle if necessary.) Yet the practice of ectogenesis would be incompatible with the *further* respect owed to our humanity on account of *the bonds of lineage, kinship and descent.* To be human means not only to have human form and powers; it means also to have a human context and to be humanly connected. The navel, no less than speech and the upright posture, is a mark of our being. It is for these sorts of reasons that we find the Brave New World's hatcheries dehumanizing.

## *Lineage and Parenthood,*
## *Embodiment and Gender*

In the summer of 1978, Louise Brown, the first human being to be conceived via *in vitro* fertilization, was born in England. Many people rejoiced at her birth. Some were pleased by the technical accomplishment, many were pleased that she was born apparently in good health. But most of us shared the joy of her parents, who after a long, frustrating and fruitless period, at last had the pleasure and

---

growing knowledge about fetal development and, especially, sophisticated procedures for performing surgery on the intrauterine fetus, even in the second trimester. Also, because viability is, in part, a matter of available outside support, technical advances—such as an artificial placenta or even less spectacular improvements in sustaining premature infants—will reveal that viability is a movable boundary and that development is a continuum without clear natural discontinuities.

blessing of a child of their own. (Curiously, the perspective of the child was largely ignored. It will thus be easier to come at the matter of lineage by looking at it first from the side of the progenitors rather than the descendants.) In the succeeding twenty-four years, thousands of people have rejoiced as did the Browns, blessed at last with a child of their own thanks only to the hand of science and technology. The desire to have a child of one's own is acknowledged to be a powerful and deep-seated human desire—some have called it instinctive—and the satisfaction of this desire, by the relief of infertility, is said to be one major goal of continuing work with *in vitro* fertilization and embryo transfer. That this is a worthy goal few, if any, would deny.

Yet let us explore what is meant by "to have a child of one's own." First, what is meant by "to have"? Is the crucial meaning that of gestating and bearing? Or is it to have as a possession? Or is it to nourish and to rear, the child being the embodiment of one's activity as teacher and guide? Or is it rather to provide someone who descends and comes after, someone who will replace oneself in the family line or preserve the family tree by new sproutings and branchings, someone who will renew and perpetuate the vitality and aspiration of human life?

More significantly, what is meant by "one's own"? What sense of the phrase is important? A scientist might define "one's own" in terms of carrying one's own genes. Though in some sense correct, this cannot be humanly decisive. For Mr. Brown or for most of us, it would not be a matter of indifference if the sperm used to fertilize the egg were provided by an identical twin brother—whose genes would be, of course, the same as his. Rather, the humanly crucial sense of one's own, the sense that leads most people to choose their own, rather than to adopt, is captured in such phrases as "my seed," "flesh of my flesh," "sprung from my loins." More accurately, since one's own is not the own of one but of two, the desire to have a child of one's own is a *couple's* desire to embody, out of the conjugal union of their separate bodies, a child who is flesh of their separate flesh made one. This archaic language may sound quaint, but I would argue that this is precisely what is being celebrated by most people who rejoice at the birth of Louise Brown, whether they would articulate it this way or not. Mr. and Mrs. Brown, by the birth of their daughter, embody themselves in another, and thus fulfill this aspect of their separate sexual natures and of their married life together. They also acquire descendants and a new branch of their joined family tree. Correlatively, the child, Louise, is given solid and unambiguous roots from which she has sprung and by which she will be nourished.

If this were to be the only use made of embryo transfer, and if providing *in this sense* "a child of one's own" were indeed the sole reason for the clinical use of the techniques, there could be no objection. Here indeed is the natural and proper home for the human embryo. Here indeed is the affirmation of transmission and the importance of lineage and connectedness. Yet there are also other uses, involving third parties, to satisfy the desire to have a child of one's own in different senses of "to have" and "one's own." I am not merely speculating about future possibilities. With the technology to effect human *in vitro* fertilization and embryo transfer has come the immediate possibility of egg donation (egg from donor, sperm from husband), embryo donation (egg and sperm from outside of the marriage), and foster pregnancy (host surrogate for gestation). Clearly, the need for extramarital embryo transfers is real and large, probably eventually even greater than that for intramarital ones.

Nearly everyone agrees that these circumstances are morally and perhaps psychologically more complicated than the intramarital ones. The reasons touch the central core of gestation and generation. Here the meaning of "one's own" is no longer so unambiguous; neither is the meaning of motherhood and the status of pregnancy. Indeed, one of the clearest meanings of having life in the laboratory is the rupture of the normally necessary umbilical connection between mother and child. This technical capacity to disrupt the connection has in fact been welcomed, curiously, for contradictory reasons. On the one hand, it is argued that embryo donation, or prenatal adoption, is superior to present adoption, precisely because the woman can have the experience of pregnancy and the child gets to be born of the adopting mother, rendering the maternal tie that much closer. On the other hand, the mother-child bond rooted in pregnancy and delivery is held to be of little consequence by those who would endorse the use of surrogate gestational mothers, say for a woman whose infertility is due to uterine disease rather than ovarian disease or oviduct obstruction. But in both cases, the new techniques serve not to ensure and preserve lineage, but rather to confound and complicate it. The principle truly at work in bringing life into the laboratory is not to provide married couples with a child of their own—or to provide a home of their own for children—but to provide a child to anyone who wants one, by whatever possible or convenient means.

So what? it will be asked. First of all, we already practice and encourage adoption. Second, we have permitted artificial insemination—though we have, after roughly fifty years of this practice, yet to resolve questions of legitimacy. Third, what with the high rate of divorce and remarriage, identification of mother, father and child are already complicated. Fourth, there is a growing rate of illegitimacy and husbandless parentages. Fifth, the use of surrogate mothers for foster pregnancy is becoming widespread with the aid of artificial insemination. Finally, our age in its enlightenment is no longer so certain about the virtues of family, lineage and heterosexuality, or even about the taboos against adultery and incest. Against this background it will be asked, Why all the fuss about some little embryos that stray from their nest?

It is not an easy question to answer. Yet consider: We practice adoption because there are abandoned children who need good homes. We do not, and would not, encourage people deliberately to generate children for others to adopt, partly because we wish to avoid baby markets, partly because we think it unfair to deliberately deprive the child of his natural ties. Recent years have seen a rise in our concern with roots, against the rootless and increasingly homogeneous background of contemporary American life. Adopted children, in particular, are pressing for information regarding their biological parents, and some states now require this information to be made available (on that typically modern rationale of freedom of information, rather than because of the far more profound importance of lineage for self-identity). Even the importance of children's ties to grandparents is being reasserted, as courts are granting visitation privileges to grandparents, over the objections of divorced-and-remarried former daughters- or sons-in-law. The practice of artificial insemination has yet to be evaluated, the secrecy in which it is practiced being an apparent concession to the dangers of publicity.* Indeed, most physicians who practice artificial insemination (donor) routinely mix in some semen from the husband, to preserve some doubt about paternity—again, a concession to the importance of lineage and legitimacy. Finally, what about the changing mores of marriage, divorce, single-parent families and sexual behavior? Do we applaud these changes? Do we want to contribute further to this confusion of thought, identity and practice?**

Our society is dangerously close to losing its grip on the meaning of some fundamental aspects of human existence. In reviewing the problem of the disrespect shown to embryonic and fetal life in our efforts to master them, we noted a tendency—we shall meet it again shortly—to reduce certain aspects of humanness to mere body, a tendency opposed most decisively in the nearly universal prohibition of cannibalism. Here, in noticing our growing casualness about marriage, legitimacy, kinship and lineage, we discover how our individualistic and willful projects lead us to ignore the truths defended by the equally widespread prohibition of incest (especially parent-child incest). Properly understood, the largely universal taboo against incest, and also the prohibitions against adultery, defend the integrity of marriage, kinship and especially the lines of origin and descent. These time-honored restraints implicitly teach that clarity about who your parents are, clarity in the lines of generation, clarity about

---

*There are today numerous suits pending, throughout the United States, because of artificial insemination with donor semen (AID). Following divorce, the ex-husbands are refusing child support for AID children, claiming, minimally, no paternity, or maximally, that the child was the fruit of an adulterous "union." In fact, a few states still treat AID as adultery. The importance of anonymity is revealed in the following bizarre case: A woman wanted to have a child, but abhorred the thought of marriage or of sexual relations with men. She learned a do-it-yourself technique of artificial insemination and persuaded a male acquaintance to donate his semen. Ten years after this virgin birth, the semen donor went to court, suing for visitation privileges to see his son.

**To those who point out that the bond between sexuality and procreation has already been effectively and permanently cleaved by the Pill, and that this is therefore an idle worry in the case of in vitro fertilization, it must be said that the Pill—like earlier forms of contraception—provides only sex without babies. Babies without sex is the truly unprecedented and radical departure.

who is whose, are the indispensable foundations of a sound family life, itself the sound foundation of civilized community. Clarity about your origins is crucial for self-identity, itself important for self-respect. It would be, in my view, deplorable public policy to erode further such fundamental beliefs, values, institutions and practices. This means, concretely, no encouragement of embryo adoption or especially of surrogate pregnancy. While it would perhaps be foolish to try to proscribe or outlaw such practices, it would not be wise to support or foster them.

The existence of human life in the laboratory, outside the confines of the generating bodies from which it sprang, also challenges the meaning of our embodiment. People like Mr. and Mrs. Brown, who seek a child derived from their flesh, celebrate in so doing their self-identification with their own bodies and acknowledge the meaning of the living human body by following its pointings to its own perpetuation. For them, their bodies contain the seeds of their own self-transcendence and enable them to strike a blow for the enduring goodness of the life in which they participate. Affirming the gift of their embodied life, they show their gratitude by passing on that gift to their children. Only the body's failure to serve the transmission of embodiment has led them—and only temporarily—to generate beyond its confines. But life in the laboratory also allows other people—including those who would donate or sell sperm, eggs or embryos; or those who would bear another's child in surrogate pregnancy; or even those who will prefer to have their children rationally manufactured entirely in the laboratory—to declare themselves independent of their bodies, in this ultimate liberation. For them the body is a mere tool, ideally an instrument of the conscious will, the sole repository of human dignity. Yet this blind assertion of will against our bodily nature—in contradiction of the meaning of the human generation it seeks to control—can only lead to self-degradation and dehumanization.

In this connection, the case of surrogate wombs bears a further comment. While expressing no objection to the practice of foster pregnancy itself, some people object that it will be done for pay, largely because of their fear that poor women will be exploited by such a practice. But if there were nothing wrong with foster pregnancy, what would be wrong with making a living at it? Clearly, this objection harbors a tacit understanding that to bear another's child for pay is in some sense a degradation of oneself—in the same sense that prostitution is a degradation primarily because it entails the loveless surrender of one's body to serve another's lust, and only derivatively because the prostitute is paid. It is to deny the meaning and worth of one's body to treat it as a mere incubator, divested of its human meaning. It is also to deny the meaning of the bonds among sexuality, love and procreation. The buying and selling of human flesh and the dehumanized uses of the human body ought not to be encouraged. To be sure, the practice of womb donation could be engaged in for love rather than for money, as it apparently has been in some cases, including the original case in Michigan. A woman could bear her sister's child out of sisterly love. But to the degree that she escapes in this way from the degradation and difficulties of the sale of human flesh and bodily services and the treating of the body as undignified stuff, once again she approaches instead the difficulties of incest and near incest.

To this point we have been examining the meaning of the presence of human life in the laboratory, but we have neglected the meaning of putting it there in the first place, that is, the meaning of extracorporeal fertilization *as such*. What is the significance of divorcing human generation from human sexuality, precisely for the meaning of our bodily natures as male and female, as both gendered and engendering? To be male or to be female derives its deepest meaning only in relation to the other, and therewith in the gender-mated prospects for generation through union. Our separated embodiment prevents us as lovers from attaining that complete fusion of souls that we as lovers seek; but the complementarity of gender provides a bodily means for transcending separateness through the children born of sexual union. As the navel is our bodily mark of lineage, pointing back to our ancestors, so our genitalia are the bodily mark of linkage, pointing ultimately forward to our descendants. Can these aspects of our being be fulfilled through the rationalized techniques of laboratory sexuality and fertilization? Does not the scientist-partner produce a triangle that somehow subverts the meaning of "two"? Even in the best of cases, when technique comes merely to the aid of our sexual natures and our marital hopes, could we be paying in coin of our humanity—whether we recognize it or not—for electing to generate sexlessly?

## Future Prospects

Before proceeding to look at some questions of public policy, we need first to consider the likely future developments regarding human life in the laboratory. In my view, we must consider these prospects in reaching our decision about present policy. For clearly, part of the meaning of what we are now doing consists in the things it will enable us, sooner or later, to do hereafter.

What can we expect for life in the laboratory, as an outgrowth of present studies? To be sure, prediction is difficult. One can never know with certainty what will happen, much less how soon. Yet uncertainty is not the same as simple ignorance. Some things, indeed, seem likely. They seem likely because (1) they are thought necessary or desirable, at least by some researchers and their sponsors; (2) they are probably biologically possible and technically feasible; and (3) they will be difficult to prevent or control (especially if no one anticipates their development or sees a need to worry about them). Wise policymakers will want to face up to reasonable projections of future accomplishments, consider whether they are cause for social concern, and see whether or not the principles now enunciated and the practices now established are adequate to deal with any such concerns. I project at least the following:

First, the growth of human embryos in the laboratory will be extended beyond the blastocyst stage. Such growth must be deemed desirable under all the arguments advanced for developmental research up to the blastocyst stage; research on gene action and regulation, epigenetic modification, chromosome segregation, cellular and organic differentiation, fetus-environment interaction, implantation and so on cannot answer all its questions with the blastocyst. Similarly, therapeutic goals that make the undifferentiated stem cells so attractive will make differentiated embryonic tissues and embryonic organs even more attractive, and we can expect enormous efforts to find ways to support embryonic growth in the laboratory to stages when these materials could be obtained. Such *in vitro* post-blastocyst differentiation has apparently been achieved in the mouse, in culture; and efforts are being made to engineer artificial placentas and wombs someday usable to support human embryological growth and development. Besides, one need not wait for such artifices: the use of other mammals as temporary hosts for human embryos is already an available possibility. How far such embryos will eventually be perpetuated is anybody's guess, but full-term ectogenesis cannot be excluded. Neither can the existence of laboratories filled with many living human embryos, growing at various stages of development.

Second, experiments will be undertaken to alter the cellular and genetic composition of these embryos, at first without subsequent transfer to a woman for gestation, perhaps later as a prelude to reproductive efforts. Again, scientific reasons now justifying current research already justify further embryonic manipulations, including formations of hybrids or chimeras (within species and between species); gene, chromosome and plasmid insertion, excision or alteration; nuclear transplantation or cloning; and so forth. In assisted-reproduction clinics, embryos are already being tested for the presence of abnormal genes and chromosomes prior to implantation ("pre-implantation genetic diagnosis"), and we may expect sooner rather than later the possibility of genetic intervention to add, subtract or alter the embryonic DNA. Techniques of DNA recombination, knowledge of the human genome and perfected skills of handling human embryos make prospects for precise genetic manipulation much nearer than anyone would have guessed ten years ago. And embryological and cellular research in mammals is making astounding progress, much of it presumably transferable to humans.*

Third, the growth of commercial and industrial-scale "human embryonics" is extremely likely. Storage and banking of living human ova and embryos have already been undertaken, complementing the commercial sperm banks established a generation ago. Dozens of biotech companies are already working on human embryos, and the products they are making—including embryos created or modified using genetic engineering—are being submitted for patents.

---

*The shape of the future was heralded back in the 1970s when the cover of *Science* featured a picture of a hexaparental mouse, born after reaggregation of an early embryo with cells disaggregated from three separate embryos. That sober journal called this a "handmade mouse"—literally a *manu-factured* mouse—and went on to say that it was "manufactured by genetic engineering techniques."

I can here do no more than identify a few kinds of questions that must be considered in relation to such possible coming control over human heredity and reproduction: questions about the wisdom required to engage in such practices; questions about the goals and standards that will guide our interventions; questions about changes in the concepts of being human, including embodiment, gender, love, lineage, identity, parenthood and sexuality; questions about the responsibility of power over future generations; questions about awe, respect, humility; questions about the kind of society we will have if we follow along our present course.

Though I cannot discuss these questions now, I can and must face a serious objection to considering them at all. Most people would agree that the projected possibilities raise far more serious questions than do simple fertilization of a few embryos, their growth *in vitro* to the blastocyst stage, and their subsequent use in experimentation or possible transfer to women for gestation. Why burden present policy with these possibilities? Future abuses, it is often said, do not disqualify present uses (though these same people also often say that "future benefits justify present practices, even questionable ones"). Moreover, there can be no certainty that A will lead to B. This thin-edge-of-the-wedge (or "slippery slope") argument has been open to criticism.

But such criticism misses the point for two reasons. First, critics often misunderstand the wedge argument, which is not primarily an argument of prediction, that A will lead to B, say, on the strength of the empirical analysis of precedent and an appraisal of the likely direction of present research. It is primarily an argument about the logic of justification. Do not the principles now used to justify the current research proposal already justify *in advance* the further developments? Consider some of these principles:

1. It is desirable to learn as much as possible about the processes of fertilization, growth, implantation and differentiation of human embryos and about human gene expression and its control.

2. It would be desirable to acquire improved techniques for enhancing conception, for preventing conception and implan-

tation, for the treatment of genetic and chromosomal abnormalities, and so on.

3. It would be desirable to extract stem cells or to harvest embryonic tissues for use in regenerative medicine.
4. In the end, only research using *human* embryos can answer these questions and provide these techniques.
5. There should be no censorship or limitation of scientific inquiry or research.

This logic knows no boundary at the blastocyst stage, or, for that matter, at any later stage. For these principles *not* to justify future extensions of current work, some independent additional principles (for example, a principle limiting such justification to particular stages of development) would have to be found. (Here, the task is to find such a biologically defensible distinction that could be respected as reasonable and not arbitrary, which is difficult—perhaps impossible—given the continuity of development after fertilization.) Perhaps even more important than any present decision to encourage bringing human life into the laboratory will be the reasons given to support that decision. We will want to know *precisely* what grounds our policymakers will give for endorsing such research, and whether their principles have not already sanctioned future developments. If they do give such wedge-opening justifications, let them do so deliberately, candidly and intentionally.

A better case to illustrate the wedge logic is the principle offered for the embryo transfer procedure as treatment for infertility. Will we support the use of *in vitro* fertilization and embryo transfer because it provides a child of one's own, in a strict sense of "one's own," to a married couple? Or will we support the transfer because it is treatment of involuntary infertility, which deserves treatment in or out of marriage, hence endorsing the use of any available technical means that would produce a healthy and normal child, including surrogate wombs, cloning or even ectogenesis?

Second, logic aside, the opponents of the wedge argument do not counsel well. It would be simply foolish to ignore what might come next and fail to make the best possible assessment of the implications of present action (or inaction). Let me put the matter bluntly:

The decisions we must now make may very well help to determine whether human beings will eventually be produced in laboratories. I say this not to shock—and I do not mean to beg the question of whether that would be desirable or not. I say this to make sure that we and our policymakers face squarely the full import and magnitude of this decision. Once the genies let the babies into the bottle, it may be impossible to get them out again.

## The Question of Federal Funding

So much, then, for the meanings of initiating, housing and manipulating human embryos in the laboratory. We are now better prepared to consider the original practical question: Should we allow or encourage these activities? The foregoing reflections still make me doubt the wisdom of proceeding with these practices, both in research and in their clinical application, notwithstanding that valuable knowledge might be had by continuing the research and identifiable suffering might be alleviated by using it to circumvent infertility. To doubt the wisdom of going ahead makes one at least a fellow traveler of the opponents of such research, but it does not, either logically or practically, require that one join them in trying to prevent it, say, by legal prohibition. Not every folly can or should be legislated against. Attempts at prohibition here would seem to be both ineffective and dangerous—ineffective because impossible to enforce; dangerous because the costs of such precedent-setting interference with scientific research might be greater than the harm it prevents. To be sure, we already have legal restrictions on experimentation with human subjects, restrictions that are manifestly not incompatible with the progress of medical science. Neither is it true that science cannot survive if it must take some direction from the law. Nor is it the case that all research, because it is research, is or should be absolutely protected. But it does not seem to me that *in vitro* fertilization and growth of human embryos or embryo transfer deserve, at least at present, to be treated as sufficiently dangerous for legislative interference.*

---

*I regard human cloning as a different matter, and favor legislative proscription. See Chapter Five.

But if doubting the wisdom does not oblige one to seek to outlaw the folly, neither does a decision to permit require a decision to encourage or support. A researcher's freedom to do *in vitro* fertilization, or a woman's right to have a child with laboratory assistance, in no way implies a public (or even a private) obligation to pay for such research or treatment. A right *against* interference is not an entitlement *for* assistance. The question repeatedly debated from 1975 through 2001 was not whether such research should be permitted or outlawed, but only whether the federal government should fund it.

I propose to discuss this policy question here, and at some length, not because it is itself timely or relatively important—it is neither—but because it is exemplary. Policy questions regarding controversial new biomedical technologies and practices—as well as other morally and politically charged matters on the border between private and public life (for example, abortion, racial discrimination, developing the artificial heart, or affirmative action)—frequently take the form of arguments over federal support. Social control and direction of new developments is often given not in terms of yes or no, but rather, how much, how fast, or how soon? Thus, much of the present analysis can be generalized and made applicable to other specific developments in the field and to the field as a whole.

The arguments in favor of federal support are well known. First, the research is seen as continuous with, if not quite an ordinary instance of, the biomedical research that the federal government supports handsomely; roughly one-half of the money spent on biomedical research in the United States comes from Uncle Sam. Why is this research different from all other research? Its scientific merit has been attested to by the normal peer review process of NIH. For some, that is a sufficient reason to support it.

Second, there are specific and highly desired practical fruits expected from the anticipated successes of this new line of research. Besides relief for many cases of infertility, the research promises new birth control measures based upon improved understanding of the mechanisms of fertilization and implantation, which in turn could lead to techniques for blocking these processes. Also, studies on early embryonic development hold forth the promise of learning how to prevent some congenital malformations and certain highly malignant tumors (for example, hydatidiform mole) that derive from aberrant fetal tissue. Most important, research with embryonic stem cells and other more developed embryonic tissues offers great hope for treatment of many serious chronic diseases and disabilities, ushering in a new era of "regenerative medicine."

Third, as he who pays the piper calls the tune, federal support would make easy federal regulation and supervision of this research. For the government to abstain, so the argument runs, is to leave the control of research and clinical application in the hands of greedy, adventurous, insensitive, reckless or power-hungry private physicians, scientists or drug companies, or, on the other hand, at the mercy of the vindictive, mindless and superstitious civic groups that will interfere with this research through state and local legislation. Only through federal regulation—which, it is said, can follow only with federal funding—will we have reasonable, enforceable and uniform guidelines.

Fourth is the chauvinistic argument that the United States should lead the way in this brave new research, especially as it will apparently be going forward in other nations. Years ago, one witness testifying before the Ethics Advisory Board that was charged to advise HEW regarding federal funding of *in vitro* fertilization research deplored the fact that the first test-tube baby was British and not American. He complained, in effect, that the existing moratorium on federal support had already created what one might call an "*in vitro* fertilization gap." Similar arguments were heard during the stem cell funding debate in 2001. The preeminence of American science and technology (and commerce!), so the argument implies, is the center of our preeminence among the nations, a position that will be jeopardized if we hang back out of fear.

Let me respond to these arguments, in reverse order. Conceding—even embracing—the premise of the importance of science for American strength and prestige, it is far from clear that failure to support *this* research would jeopardize American science. Certainly the use of embryo transfer to overcome infertility, though a vital matter for the couples involved, is hardly a matter of vital national interest—at least not unless and until the majority of American women are similarly infertile. The demands of international competition, admittedly often a necessary evil, should be invoked only for things that really matter; a missile gap and an embryo transfer gap are chasms apart. In areas not crucial to our own survival, there will be many things we should allow other nations to develop, if that is their wish, without feeling obliged to join them. Moreover, one should not rush into potential folly in order to avoid being the last to commit it.

The argument about governmental regulation has much to recommend it. But it fails to consider that there are other safeguards against recklessness, at least in the clinical applications, known to the high-minded as the canons of medical ethics and to the cynical as liability for malpractice. Also, federal regulations attached to federal funding will not in any case regulate research done with private monies, for example, by the drug companies. Moreover, there are enough concerned practitioners of these new arts who would have a compelling interest in regulating their own practice, if only to escape the wrath and interference of hostile citizens' groups in response to unsavory goings-on. Organized professional societies have and will issue guidelines for their members, and the prestige of membership keeps even the more adventurous from violating the norms. The available evidence does not convince me that a sensible practice of *in vitro* experimentation requires regulation by the federal government.

In turning to the argument about anticipated technological powers, we face difficult calculations of unpredictable and more-or-less likely costs and benefits, and the all-important questions of priorities in the allocation of scarce resources. Here it seems useful to consider separately the techniques for generating children, the anticipated techniques for birth control or for preventing developmental anomalies and malignancies, and studies that could usher in the great age of regenerative medicine.

First, accepting that providing a child of their own to infertile couples is a worthy goal—and it is both insensitive and illogical to cite the population problem as an argument for ignoring the problem of infertility—one can nevertheless question its rank relative to other goals of medical research. One can even wonder whether it is indeed a *medical* goal, or a worthy goal for medicine, that is, whether alleviating infertility, especially in this way, is part of the art of healing. Just as abortion for genetic defect is a peculiar innovation in medicine (or in preventive medicine) in which a disease is treated by eliminating the patient (or, if you prefer, a disease is prevented by "preventing" the patient), so laboratory fertilization is a peculiar treatment for oviduct obstruction in that it requires the creation of a new life to "heal" an existing one. All this simply emphasizes the uniqueness of the reproductive organs in that their proper function involves other people, and calls attention to the fact that infertility is not a disease, like heart disease or stroke, even though obstruction of a normally patent tube or vessel is the proximate cause of each.

However this may be, there is a more important objection to this approach to the problem. It represents yet another instance of our thoughtless preference for expensive, high-technology, therapy-oriented approaches to disease and dysfunctions. What about spending this money on discovering the causes of infertility? What about the prevention of tubal obstruction? We complain about rising medical costs, but we insist on the most spectacular and the most technological—and thereby often the most costly—remedies.

The truth is that we do know a little about the causes of tubal obstruction, though much less than we should or could. For instance, it is estimated that at least one-third of such cases are the aftermath of pelvic inflammatory disease, caused by that uninvited venereal guest, gonococcus. Leaving aside any question about whether it makes sense for a federally funded baby to be the wage of aphrodisiac indiscretion, one can only look with wonder at a society that will have "petri-dish babies"* before it has found a vaccine against gonorrhea.

True, there are other causes of blocked oviducts, and blocked oviducts are not the only cause of female infertility. True, it is not logically necessary to choose between prevention and cure. But *practically*

---

*There has been much objection, largely from the scientific community, to the phrase "test-tube baby." More than one commentator has deplored the exploitation of its "flesh-creeping" connotations. They point out that a flat petri dish is used, not a test tube—as if that mattered—and that the embryo spends only a few days in the dish. But they don't ask why the term "test-tube baby" remains the popular designation, and whether it does not embody more of the deeper truth than a more accurate, laboratory appellation. If the decisive difference is between "in the womb" or "in the lab,"

speaking, with money for research as limited as it is, federal research funds targeted for the relief of infertility should certainly go first to epidemiological and preventive measures—especially where the costs of success in the high-technology cure are likely to be great.

What about these costs? I have already explored some of the nonfinancial costs, in discussing the meaning of the research for our images of humanness. Let us, for now, consider only the financial costs. How expensive is a baby produced with the aid of *in vitro* fertilization? Hard to say exactly. To the costs of hormone preparation of ovaries and uterus, laparoscopy, fertilization and growth *in vitro*, and transfer, one must add the costs of closely monitoring the baby's development to check on her "normality" and, should it come, the costs of governmental regulation. And then there are the costs of failure and having to try again. A conservative estimate places the costs of a successful pregnancy of this kind between $10,000 and $15,000. If we use the conservative figure of 500,000 for estimating the number of infertile women with blocked oviducts in the United States whose *only* hope of having children lies with *in vitro* fertilization,* we reach a conservative estimate cost of $5 to $7.5 billion. Is it fiscally wise for the federal government to start down this road?

Clearly not, if it is also understood that the costs of providing the service, rendered possible by a successful technology, will also

---

the popular designation conveys it (see "An Afterword," below). And it is right on target, and puts us on notice, if the justification for the present laboratory procedures tacitly also justifies future extensions, including full ectogenesis, say, if that were the only way a wombless woman could have a child of her own, without renting a human womb from a surrogate bearer.

*This figure is calculated from estimates that between 10 and 15 percent of all couples are involuntarily infertile, and that in more than half of these cases the cause is in the female. Blocked oviducts account for perhaps 20 percent of the causes of female infertility. Perhaps 50 percent of these women might be helped to have a child by means of reconstructive surgery on the oviducts; the remainder could conceive *only* with the aid of laboratory fertilization and embryo transfer. These estimates do not include additional candidates with uterine disease (who could "conceive" only by embryo transfer to surrogate-gestators), nor those with ovarian dysfunction who would need egg donation as well, nor that growing population of women who have had tubal ligations and who could later turn to *in vitro* fertilization. It is also worth noting that not all the infertile couples are childless; indeed, a surprising number are seeking to enlarge an existing family.

be borne by the taxpayers. Nearly everyone now agrees that the kidney machine legislation, obliging the federal government to pay for kidney dialysis for anyone in need, is an impossible precedent—notwithstanding that individual lives have been prolonged as a result. But once the technique of *in vitro* fertilization and embryo transfer is developed and available, how should the baby-making be paid for? Should it be covered under medical insurance? If a national health insurance program is enacted, will and should these services be included? (Those who argue that they are part of medicine will have a hard time saying no.) Failure to do so will make this procedure available only to the well-to-do, on a fee-for-service basis. Would that be a fair alternative? Perhaps, but it is unlikely to be tolerated. Indeed, the principle of equality—equal access to equal levels of medical care—is the leading principle in the press for medical reform. One can be certain that efforts will be forthcoming to make this procedure available equally to all, independent of ability to pay, under Medicaid or national health insurance or in some other way. (A few years ago, an egalitarian Boston-based group concerned with infertility managed to obtain private funding to pay for artificial insemination for women on welfare!)

Much as I sympathize with the plight of infertile couples, I do not believe they are entitled to the provision of a child at public expense, especially now, especially at this cost, especially by a procedure that also involves so many moral difficulties. Given the many vexing dilemmas that will surely be spawned by laboratory-assisted reproduction, the federal government should not be misled by compassion to embark on this imprudent course.

In considering the federal funding of such research for its other anticipated technological benefits, independent of its clinical use in baby-making, we face a more difficult matter. In brief, as is the case with all basic research, one simply cannot predict what kinds of techniques and uses it will yield. But here, also, I think good sense would at present say that before one undertakes human *in vitro* fertilization to seek new methods of birth control (for example, by developing antibodies to the human egg that would physically interfere with its fertilization) one should make adequate attempts to do this in animals. One simply can't get sufficient numbers of human eggs to do this pioneering research well—at least not without subjecting countless women to additional risks not to their immediate benefit. Why not test this conceit first in the mouse or rabbit? Only if the results were very promising—and judged also to be relatively safe in practice—should one consider trying such things in humans. Likewise, the developmental research can and should be first carried out in animals, especially in primates. Purely on scientific grounds, the federal government ought not *now* to be investing its funds in this research for its promised technological benefits—benefits that, in the absence of pilot studies in animals, must be regarded as mere wishful thoughts in the imaginings of scientists.

The use of human embryos for stem cell research, the current subject of controversy, is a much closer call. Proponents of this research believe that it carries enormous benefits for millions who now suffer from incurable diseases and disabilities—orders of magnitude greater than the numbers of infertile couples—through regenerative medicine. This is today a most fashionable area of research, and although no one knows whether it will pay off, it would be foolish to gainsay it. Debate continues as to whether embryonic stem cells will be more or less effective than adult (or nonembryonic) stem cells in the treatment of disease; but as of this writing there is no evidence that tissues derived from embryonic stem cells have produced a true cure of any human disease, even in animal models of human diseases. Privately funded stem cell research will certainly proceed. Thanks to President Bush's decision, federal funds are available now for work on some sixty-four embryonic stem cell lines established before that decision was made. We are a long way from knowing whether this research will succeed and whether any more cell lines will be needed. But before we face this question, every effort should be made both to exploit the potential of adult stem cells and to prove that embryonic stem cell treatments can actually cure diseases in animals.

There remains the first justification: research for the sake of knowledge itself—knowledge about cell cleavage, cell-cell and cell-environment interactions, and cell differentiation; knowledge of gene action and gene regulation in both normal and diseased tissues; knowledge of normal and abnormal embryonic development; knowledge of the effects and mechanisms of the action of various chemical and physical agents on growth and development; knowledge of the basic processes of fertilization and implantation. This is all knowledge worth having, and though much can be learned using animal sources—and these sources have barely begun to be sufficiently exploited—the investigation of these matters in *man* would, sooner or later, require the use of human embryonic material. Here, again, there are questions of research priority about which there is room for disagreement, among scientists and laymen alike. But there is also a more fundamental matter.

Is such research consistent with the ethical standards of our community? The question turns in large part on the status of the early human embryo. If, as I have argued, the early embryo is deserving of respect because of what it is, now and potentially, it is difficult to justify submitting it to invasive experiments, and especially difficult to justify *creating* it solely for the purpose of experimentation. The reader should test this conclusion against his or her reaction to imagining the Fertilizing Room of the Central London Hatchery or, more modestly, to encountering an incubator or a refrigerator full of living embryos.

But even if this argument fails to sway our policymakers, another one should. For their decision, I remind you, is not whether *in vitro* fertilization and embryo research should be permitted in the United States, but whether our tax dollars should encourage and foster it. One cannot, therefore, ignore the deeply held convictions of a sizable portion of our population—it may even be a majority—that regards the human embryo as protectable humanity, not to be experimented upon except for its own benefit. Never mind if these beliefs have a religious foundation—as if that should ever be a reason for dismissing them! The presence, sincerity and depth of these beliefs, and the grave importance of their subject, are what must concern us. The holders of these beliefs have been very much alienated by the numerous court decisions and legislative enactments regarding abortion and research on fetuses. Many who by and large share their opinions about the humanity of prenatal life have with heavy heart gone along with the liberalization of abortion, out of deference to the wishes, desires, interests or putative rights of pregnant women. But will they go along with what they can only regard as gratuitous and willful assaults on human life, or at least on potential and salvageable human life, and on human dignity? We can ill afford to alienate them further, and it would be unstatesmanlike, to say the least, to do so, especially in a matter so full of potential dangers.

Technological progress is but one measure of our national health. Far more important is the affection and esteem in which our citizenry holds its laws and institutions. No amount of relieved infertility is worth the further disaffection and civil contention that the lifting of the moratorium on federal funding is likely to produce. People opposed to abortion and people willing to permit women to obtain elective abortion but at their own expense will not tolerate having their tax money spent on scientific research that requires what they consider to be cruelty at best, and possibly murder. Wise statesmanship will take this matter most seriously and continue to refuse to lift the moratorium on federal funding of embryo research— at least until persuaded that the public will give its overwhelming support. Imprudence in this matter may be the worst sin of all.

## An Afterword

This has been for me a long and difficult exposition. Many of the arguments are hard to make. It is hard to get confident people to face unpleasant prospects. It is hard to ask people to take seriously such "soft" matters as lineage, identity, respect and self-respect when they are in tension with such "hard" matters as a cure for infertility or new methods of contraception. It is hard to claim respect for human life in the laboratory in a society that does not respect human life in the womb. It is hard to talk about the meaning of sexuality and embodiment in a culture that treats sex increasingly as sport and has trivialized gender, marriage and procreation. It is hard to oppose federal funding of baby making in a society that increasingly expects the federal government to satisfy all demands, and that—contrary to so much evidence of waste, incompetence and corruption—continues to believe that only Uncle Sam can do it. And, finally, it is hard to speak about restraint in a culture that seems to venerate very little above man's own attempt to master all. Here, I am afraid, is the biggest question about the reasonableness of the desire to become masters and possessors of nature, human nature included.

Here we approach the deepest meaning of *in vitro* fertilization. Those who have likened it to artificial insemination are only partly correct. With *in vitro* fertilization, the human embryo emerges for the first time from the natural darkness and privacy of its mother's womb, where it is hidden away in mystery, into the bright light and utter publicity of the scientist's laboratory, where it will be treated with unswerving rationality, before the clever and shameless eye of the mind and beneath the obedient and equally clever touch of the hand. What does it mean to hold the beginning of human life before your eyes, in your hands—even for five days (for the meaning does not depend on duration)? Perhaps the meaning is contained in the following story.

Long ago there was a man of great intellect and great courage. He was a remarkable man, a giant, able to answer questions that no other human being could answer, willing boldly to face any challenge or problem. He was a confident man, a masterful man. He saved his city from disaster and ruled it as a father rules his children, revered by all. But something was wrong in his city. A plague had fallen on generation; infertility afflicted plants, animals and humans. The man promised to uncover the cause of the plague and cure the infertility. Resolutely, confidently, he put his sharp mind to work to solve the problem, to bring the dark things to light. No reticence, no secrets, a full public inquiry. He raged against the representatives of caution, moderation, prudence and piety, who urged him to curtail his inquiry; he accused them of trying to usurp his rightfully earned power, to replace human and masterful control with submissive reverence. The story ends in tragedy: He solves the problem, but in making visible and public the dark and intimate details of his origins, he ruins his life and that of his family. In the end, too late, he learns about the price of presumption, of overconfidence, of the overweening desire to master and control one's fate. In symbolic rejection of his desire to look into everything, he punishes his eyes with self-inflicted blindness.

Sophocles seems to suggest that such a man is always in principle—albeit unwittingly—a patricide, a regicide and a practitioner of incest. These are the crimes of the tyrant, that misguided and vain seeker of self-sufficiency and full autonomy, who loathes being reminded of his dependence and neediness, who crushes all opposition to the assertion of his will, and whose incest is symbolic of his desire to be the godlike source of his own being. His character is his destiny.

We men of modern science may have something to learn from our philosophical forebear Oedipus. It appears that Oedipus, being the kind of man an Oedipus is (the chorus calls him a paradigm of man), had no choice but to learn through suffering. Is it really true that we, too, have no other choice?

# CHAPTER FOUR

# The Age of Genetic Technology Arrives

As one contemplates the current and projected state of genetic knowledge and technology, one is astonished by how far we have come in the less than fifty years since Watson and Crick first announced the structure of DNA. True, soon after that discovery, scientists began seriously to discuss the futuristic prospects of gene therapy for genetic disease and of genetic engineering more generally. But no one then imagined how rapidly genetic technology would emerge. The Human Genome Project, disclosing the DNA sequences of all thirty thousand human genes, is all but completed. And even without comprehensive genomic knowledge, biotech business is booming. According to a recent report by the research director for Glaxo Smith Kline, enough sequencing data are already available to keep his researchers busy for the next twenty years, developing early-detection screening techniques, rationally designed vaccines, genetically engineered changes in malignant tumors leading to enhanced immune response, and, ultimately, precise gene therapy for specific genetic diseases. The age of genetic technology has arrived.

Genetic technology comes into existence as part of the large humanitarian project to cure disease, prolong life and alleviate suffering. As such, it occupies the moral high ground of compassionate healing. Who would not welcome personal genetic profiling that would enable doctors to customize the most effective and safest drug treatments for individuals with hypertension or rheumatoid arthritis? Who would not welcome genetic therapy to correct the defects that lead to sickle cell anemia, Huntington's disease and breast cancer, or to protect against the immune deficiency caused by the AIDS virus?

And yet genetic technology has also aroused considerable public concern, for it strikes most people as different from other biomedical technologies. Even people duly impressed by the astonishing genetic achievements of the last decades and eager for the medical benefits are nonetheless ambivalent about these new developments. For they sense that genetic technology, while in some respects continuous with the traditional medical project of compassionate healing, also represents something radically new and disquieting. Often hard-pressed to articulate the precise basis of their disquiet, they talk rather in general terms about the dangers of eugenics or the fear of "tampering with human genes" or, for that matter, "playing God."

Enthusiasts for genetic technology, made confident by their expertise and by their growing prestige and power, are often impatient with the public's unease. Much of it they attribute to ignorance of science: "If the public only knew what we know, it would see things our way and give up its irrational fears." For the rest, they blame outmoded moral and religious notions, ideas that scientists insist no longer hold water and only serve to obstruct scientific progress.

In my own view, the scientists' attempt to cast the debate as a battle of beneficial and knowledgeable cleverness versus ignorant and superstitious anxiety should be resisted. For the public is right to be ambivalent about genetic technology, and no amount of instruction in molecular biology and genetics should allay its—our—legitimate human concerns. Rightly understood, these worries are, in fact, in touch with the deepest matters of our humanity and dignity, and we ignore them at our peril.

I aim to articulate some of those concerns, bearing in mind that genetic technology cannot be treated in isolation but must be seen in connection with other advances in reproductive and developmental biology, in neurobiology and in the genetics of behavior—indeed, with all the techniques now and soon being marshaled to intervene ever more directly and precisely into the bodies and minds of human beings. For the sake of this discussion, I will take the technical claims of the enthusiasts for genetic technology at face value, although I suspect that a fair number of their claims are exaggerated. Discovering the DNA sequences is far easier than learning how genes interact within the living body or what they mean, clinically speaking. Synthesizing a healthy gene to replace a defective one is much easier than delivering it safely to the right places in the body and having it work only as desired. Even the fine idea of perfected, individualized therapies based on genetic profiling is, I suspect, going to face great practical obstacles before it can be widely used, and even then, the costs of doing so may be prohibitive. Yet I will not dispute here about which of the prophesied technologies will in fact prove feasible or how soon.* To be sure, as a practical matter we must address the particular ethical issues raised by each new technical power as it comes into existence. But the moral meaning of the entire enterprise does not depend on the precise details regarding what and when. I shall proceed by raising a series of questions, the first of which is an attempt to say how genetic technology is different.

## *Is Genetic Technology Special?*

What is different about genetic technology? At first glance, not much. Isolating a disease-inducing aberrant gene looks fairly continuous with isolating a disease-inducing intracellular virus. Supplying diabetics with normal genes for producing insulin has the same medical goal as supplying them with insulin for injection.

Nevertheless, despite these obvious similarities, genetic technology is also decisively different. When fully developed, it will wield two powers not shared by ordinary medical practice. Medicine treats only existing individuals, and it treats them only remedially, seeking to correct deviations from a more or less stable norm of health. By contrast, genetic engineering will, first of all, deliberately make changes that are transmissible into succeeding generations and may even alter in advance specific *future* individuals through direct "germline" or embryo interventions. Second, genetic engineering may be able, through so-called genetic enhancement, to create new human capacities and, hence, new norms of health and fitness.**

---

*I will also not dispute here the scientists' reductive understanding of life and their treatment of rich vital activities solely in terms of the interactions of genes (and other lifeless molecules). I do, however, touch on the moral significance of such reductionism toward the end of this essay.

**Some commentators, in disagreement with these arguments, insist that genetic technology differs only in degree from previous human practices that have existed for

For the present, it is true, genetic technology is hailed primarily for its ability better to diagnose and treat *disease* in *existing* individuals. Confined to such practices, it would raise few questions (beyond the usual ones of safety and efficacy). Even intrauterine gene therapy for existing fetuses with diagnosable genetic disease could be seen as an extension of the growing field of fetal medicine.

But there is no reason to believe that the use of gene-altering powers can be so confined, either in logic or in practice. For one thing, "germ-line" gene therapy and manipulation, affecting not merely the unborn but also the unconceived,* is surely in our future. The practice has numerous justifications, beginning with the desire to reverse the unintended dysgenic effects of modern medical success. Thanks to medicine, for example, individuals who would have died from diabetes now live long enough to transmit their disease-producing genes. Why, it has been argued, should we not reverse these unfortunate changes by deliberate intervention? More generally, why should we not effect precise genetic alteration in disease-carrying sperm or eggs or early embryos, in order to prevent in

---

millennia. For example, they see no difference between the "social engineering" of education, which works on the next generation through speech or symbolic deed, and biological engineering, which inscribes its effects, directly and irreversibly, into the human constitution. Or they claim to see no difference between the indirect genetic effects of human mate selection and deliberate, direct genetic engineering to produce offspring with precise biological capacities. Such critics, I fear, have already bought into a reductionist view of human life and the relation between the generations. They speak about children not as gifts that we are duty-bound to humanize through speech and example in light of the good, but as products whose qualities we determine by manipulating their bodies, consulting only our own subjective prejudices. They fail to notice that education works through the soul, through *meanings* (necessarily immaterial) conveyed in speech and deed. And they ignore the fact that most people choose their mates for reasons different from stud farming. Though mindful of the heritable implications of choosing a spouse, people pay attention to character, tastes and the things each partner esteems and aspires to in life, not merely some morally neutral, genetically determined capacity. The former are more important than the latter for rearing *human* offspring.

*Correction of a genetically abnormal egg or sperm (that is, of the "germ cells"), however worthy an activity, stretches the meaning of "therapy" beyond all normal uses. Just who is the "patient" being "treated"? The potential child-to-be that might be formed out of such egg or sperm is, at the time of the treatment, at best no more than a hope and a hypothesis. There is no medical analogue for treatment of nonexistent patients.

advance the emergence of disease that otherwise will later require expensive and burdensome treatment? And why should not parents eager to avoid either the birth of afflicted children or the trauma of eugenic abortion be able to avail themselves of germ-line alteration? In short, even before we have had more than trivial experience with gene therapy for existing individuals—none of it successful—sober people have called for overturning the current (self-imposed) taboo on germ-line modification.[1] The line between somatic and germ-line modification cannot hold.

Despite the naive hopes of many, neither will we be able to defend the boundary between therapy and genetic enhancement. Will we reject novel additions to the human genome that enable us to produce, internally, vitamins or amino acids we now must get in our diet? Will we oppose the insertion of engineered foreign (or even animal) genes fatal to bacteria and parasites or offering us increased resistance to cancer? Will we decline to make alterations in the immune system that will increase its efficacy or make it impervious to HIV? When genetic profiling becomes able to disclose the genetic contributions to height or memory or intelligence, will we deny prospective parents the right to enhance the potential of their children?* Finally, should we discover—as no doubt we will—the genetic switches that control our biological clock and that very likely influence also the maximum human life expectancy, will we opt to keep our hands off the rate of aging or our natural human lifespan? Not a chance.

We thus face a paradox. On the one hand, genetic technology really *is* different. It can and will go to work directly and deliberately on our basic, heritable, life-shaping capacities at their biological roots. It can take us beyond existing norms of health and healing—perhaps even alter fundamental features of human nature. On the other hand, precisely because the goals it will serve, at least to begin with, will be continuous with those of modern high-

---

*To be sure, not all attempts at enhancement will require genetic alterations. We have already witnessed efforts to boost height with supplementary growth hormone or athletic performance with steroids or "blood doping." Nevertheless, the largest possible changes in what is "normally" human are likely to come about only with the help of genetic alterations or the joining of machines (for example, computers) to human beings.

interventionist medicine, we will find its promise familiar and irresistible.

This paradox itself contributes to public disquiet: rightly perceiving a powerful difference in genetic technology, we also sense that we are powerless to establish, on the basis of that difference, clear limits to its use. The genetic genie, first unbottled to treat disease, will go its own way, whether we like it or not.

## How Much Genetic Self-Knowledge Is Good for Us?

Quite apart from worries about genetic engineering, gaining genetic knowledge is itself a legitimate cause of anxiety, not least because of one of its most touted benefits—the genetic profiling of individuals. There has been much discussion about how knowledge of someone's genetic defects, if leaked to outsiders, could be damaging in terms of landing a job or gaining health or life insurance, and legislative measures have been enacted to guard against such hazards. Little attention has been paid, however, to the implications of genetic knowledge for the person himself. Yet the deepest problem connected with learning your own genetic sins and unhealthy predispositions is neither the threat to confidentiality nor the risk of "genetic discrimination" in employment or insurance, important though these practical problems may be.* It is, rather, the various hazards and deformations in living your life that will attach to knowing in advance

---

*I find it odd that it is these issues that have been put forward as the special ethical problems associated with genetic technology and the Human Genome Project. Issues of privacy and risks of discrimination related to medical conditions are entirely independent of whether the medical condition is genetic in origin. Only if a special stigma were attached to having an *inherited* disease—for example, only if having thalassemia or sickle cell anemia were more shameful than having gonorrhea or lung cancer—would the genetic character of a disease create special or additional reasons for protecting against breaches of confidentiality or discrimination in the workplace. It is, however, true that special questions of confidentiality and disclosure do arise for patients with genetic disease because, with heritable traits, a patient's relatives may be similarly afflicted; and they may arguably have a "need to know" that might put pressure on the right of privacy for the patient. Yet even here, the troubles such knowledge could produce within families go far beyond threats to privacy.

your likely or possible medical future. To be sure, in some cases such foreknowledge will be welcome, if it can lead to easy measures to prevent or treat the impending disorder, and if the disorder in question does not powerfully affect self-image or self-command. But will and should we welcome knowledge that we carry a predisposition to Alzheimer's disease, schizophrenia, or some other personality or behavior disorder, or genes that will definitely produce, at an unknown future time, a serious but untreatable disease?

Still harder will it be for most people to live easily and wisely with less certain information — say, where multigenic traits are involved or where the predictions are purely statistical, with no clear implication for any particular "predisposed" individual. The recent case of a father who insisted that ovariectomy and mastectomy be performed on his ten-year-old daughter because she happened to carry the BRCA-1 gene for breast cancer dramatically shows the toxic effect of genetic knowledge.

Less dramatic but more profound is the threat to human freedom and spontaneity, a subject explored twenty-five years ago by the philosopher Hans Jonas, one of our wisest commentators on technology and the human prospect. In a discussion of human cloning, Jonas argued for a "right to ignorance":

> That there can be (and mostly is) too little knowledge has always been realized; that there can be too much of it stands suddenly before us in a blinding light.... The ethical command here entering the enlarged stage of our powers is: never to violate the right to that ignorance which is a condition for the possibility of authentic action; or: *to respect the right of each human life to find its own way and be a surprise to itself.*[2]

To scientists convinced that their knowledge of predispositions can only lead to rational preventive medicine, Jonas's defense of ignorance will look like obscurantism. It is not. As Jonas observes, "knowledge of the future, especially one's own, has always been excepted [from the injunction to 'Know thyself'] and the attempt to gain it by whatever means (astrology is one) disparaged — as futile superstition by the enlightened, but as sin by theologians; and in the latter case with reasons that are also philosophically sound."[3] And although everyone remembers that Prometheus was the philanthropic god who gave fire and the arts to humans, it is often forgotten that he gave them also the greater gift of "blind hopes"—"to cease seeing doom before their eyes"[4]—precisely because he knew that ignorance of one's own future fate was indispensable to aspiration and achievement. I suspect that many people, taking their bearings from life lived open-endedly rather than from preventive medicine practiced rationally, would prefer ignorance of the future to the scientific astrology of knowing their genetic profile. In a free society, that would be their right.

Or would it? This leads us to the third question.

## What about Freedom?

Even people who might otherwise welcome the growth of genetic knowledge and technology are worried about the coming power of geneticists, genetic engineers and, in particular, governmental authorities armed with genetic technology.* Precisely because we have been taught by these very scientists that genes hold the secret of life, and that our genotype is our essence if not quite our destiny, we are made nervous by those whose expert knowledge and technique touch our very being. Even apart from any particular abuses and misuses of power, friends of human freedom have deep cause for concern.

C. S. Lewis, no friend of ignorance, put the matter sharply in *The Abolition of Man*:

> It is, of course, a commonplace to complain that men have hitherto used badly, and against their fellows, the powers that science has given them. But that is not the point I am trying to

---

*Until the events of September 11 and the anthrax scare that followed, they did not worry enough. It is remarkable that most bioethical discussions of genetic technology had naively neglected its potential usefulness in creating biological weapons, such as, to begin with, antibiotic-resistant plague bacteria, or, later, aerosols containing cancer-inducing or mind-scrambling viral vectors. The most outstanding molecular geneticists were especially naive in this area. When American molecular biologists convened the 1975 Asilomar Conference on recombinant DNA research, which called for a voluntary moratorium on experiments until the biohazards could be evaluated, they invited Soviet biologists to the meeting who said virtually nothing but who photographed every slide that was shown.

make. I am not speaking of particular corruptions and abuses which an increase of moral virtue would cure: I am considering what the thing called "Man's power over Nature" must always and essentially be. . . .

In reality . . . if any one age really attains, by eugenics and scientific education, the power to make its descendants what it pleases, all men who live after it are the patients of that power. They are weaker, not stronger: for though we may have put wonderful machines in their hands we have pre-ordained how they are to use them. . . . The real picture is that of one domi-nant age . . . which resists all previous ages most successfully and dominates all subsequent ages most irresistibly, and thus is the real master of the human species. But even within this mas-ter generation (itself an infinitesimal minority of the species) the power will be exercised by a minority smaller still. Man's con-quest of Nature, if the dreams of some scientific planners are realized, means the rule of a few hundreds of men over billions upon billions of men. There neither is nor can be any simple increase of power on Man's side. Each new power won *by* man is a power *over* man as well. Each advance leaves him weaker as well as stronger. In every victory, besides being the general who triumphs, he is also the prisoner who follows the triumphal car.[5]

Most genetic technologists will hardly recognize themselves in this portrait. Though they concede that abuses or misuses of power may occur, especially in tyrannical regimes, they see themselves not as predestinators but as facilitators, merely providing increased knowledge and technique that people can freely choose to use in making decisions about their health or reproductive choices. Genetic power, they tell us, serves not to limit freedom, but to increase it.

But as we can see from the already existing practices of genetic screening and prenatal diagnosis, this claim is at best self-deceptive, at worst disingenuous. The choice to develop and practice genetic screening and the choices of which genes to target for testing have been made not by the public but by scientists—and not on liberty-enhancing but on eugenic grounds. In many cases, practitioners of prenatal diagnosis refuse to do fetal genetic screening in the absence of a prior commitment from the pregnant woman to abort any afflicted fetus. In other situations, pregnant women who still wish *not* to know prenatal facts must withstand strong medical pressures for testing.

While a small portion of the population may be sufficiently educated to participate knowingly and freely in genetic decisions, most people are and will no doubt always be subject to the benevolent tyranny of expertise. Every expert knows how easy it is to get most people to choose one way rather than another simply by the way one raises the questions, describes the prognosis and presents the options. The preferences of counselors will always overtly or subtly shape the choices of the counseled.

In addition, economic pressures to contain health-care costs will almost certainly constrain free choice. Refusal to provide insurance coverage for this or that genetic disease may eventually work to compel genetic abortion or intervention. State-mandated screening already occurs for PKU (phenylketonuria) and other diseases, and full-blown genetic screening programs loom large on the horizon. Once these arrive, there will likely be an upsurge of economic pressure to limit reproductive freedom. All this will be done, of course, in the name of the well-being of children.

Already in 1971, geneticist Bentley Glass, in his presidential address to the American Association for the Advancement of Science, enunciated "the right of every child to be born with a sound physical and mental constitution, based on a sound genotype." Looking ahead to the reproductive and genetic technologies that are today rapidly arriving, Glass proclaimed: "No parents will in that future time have a right to burden society with a malformed or a mentally incompetent child."[6] It remains to be seen to what extent such prophecies will be realized. But they surely provide sufficient and reasonable grounds for being concerned about restrictions on human freedom, even in the absence of overt coercion, and even in liberal polities like our own.

## What about Human Dignity?

Here, rather than in the more-discussed fears about freedom, lie our deepest concerns, and rightly so. For threats to human dignity can—and probably will—arise even with the free, humane and "enlightened" use of these technologies. Genetic technology, the practices it will engender, and above all the scientific teachings about human life on which it rests are not, as many would have it, morally and humanly neutral. Regardless of how they are practiced or taught, they are pregnant with their own moral meaning, and will necessarily bring with them changes in our practices, our institutions, our norms, our beliefs and our self-conception. It is, I submit, these challenges to our dignity and humanity that are at the bottom of our anxiety over genetic science and technology. Let me touch briefly on four aspects of this most serious matter.

### *"Playing God"*

Paradoxically, worries about dehumanization are sometimes expressed in the fear of superhumanization, that is, that man will be "playing God." This complaint is too facilely dismissed by scientists and non-believers. The concern has meaning, God or no God. By it is meant one or more of the following: man, or *some* men, are becoming creators of life, and indeed, of individual living human beings (*in vitro* fertilization, cloning); they stand in judgment of each being's worthiness to live or die (genetic screening and abortion)—not on moral grounds, as is said of God's judgment, but on somatic and genetic ones; they also hold out the promise of salvation from our genetic sins and defects (gene therapy and genetic engineering).

Never mind the exaggeration that lurks in this conceit of man's playing God. (Even at his most powerful, after all, man is capable only of *playing* God.) Never mind the implicit innuendo that nobody has given to others this creative and judgmental authority, or the implicit retort that there is theological warrant for acting as God's co-creator in overcoming the ills and suffering of the world. Consider only that if scientists are seen in this godlike role of creator, judge and savior, the rest of us must stand before them as supplicating, tainted creatures. Despite the hyperbolic speech, that is worry enough.

Practitioners of prenatal diagnosis, working today with but a fraction of the information soon to be available from the Human Genome Project, already screen for a long list of genetic diseases and abnormalities, from Down syndrome to dwarfism. Possession of any one of these defects, they believe, renders a prospective child unworthy of life. Persons who happen still to be born with these conditions, having somehow escaped the spreading net of detection and eugenic abortion, are increasingly regarded as "mistakes," as inferior human beings who should not have been born.* Not long ago, at my own university, a physician making rounds with medical students stood over the bed of an intelligent, otherwise normal ten-year-old boy with spina bifida. "Were he to have been conceived today," the physician casually informed his entourage, "he would have been aborted." Determining who shall live and who shall die—on the basis of genetic merit—is a godlike power already wielded by genetic medicine. This power will only grow.

### Manufacture and Commodification

But, one might reply, genetic technology also holds out the promise of redemption, of a *cure* for these life-crippling and life-forfeiting disorders. Very well. But in order truly to practice their salvific power, genetic technologists will have to increase greatly their manipulations and interventions, well beyond merely screening and weeding out. True, in some cases genetic testing and risk management aimed at prevention may actually cut down on the need for high-tech interventions aimed at cure. But in many other cases, ever-greater genetic scrutiny will lead necessarily to ever more extensive manipulation. And, to produce Bentley Glass's healthy and well-endowed babies, let alone babies with the benefits of genetic enhancement, a new scientific obstetrics will be necessary, one that will come very close to turning human procreation into manufacture.

This process was already crudely begun with *in vitro* fertilization. It is now taking giant steps forward with the ability to screen *in vitro* embryos before implantation (so-called pre-implantation

---

*In the early 1970s, I tried to grapple with this issue in an essay, "Perfect Babies: Pre-Natal Diagnosis and the Equal Right to Life," which appears as Chapter Three in my book *Toward a More Natural Science: Biology and Human Affairs* (New York: The Free Press, 1985). One of the most worrisome but least appreciated aspects of the godlike power of the new genetics is its tendency to "redefine" a human being in terms of his genes. Once a person is decisively characterized by his genotype, it is but a short step to justifying death solely for genetic sins.

genetic diagnosis). And it will come to maturity with interventions such as cloning and, eventually, with precise genetic engineering. Just follow the logic and the aspirations of current practice: the road we are traveling leads all the way to the world of designer babies — reached not by dictatorial fiat, but by the march of benevolent humanitarianism, and cheered on by an ambivalent citizenry that also dreads becoming merely the last of man's manmade things.

Make no mistake: the price to be paid for producing optimum or even only genetically sound babies will be the transfer of procreation from the home to the laboratory. Increasing control over the product can only be purchased by the increasing depersonalization of the entire process and its coincident transformation into manufacture. Such an arrangement will be profoundly dehumanizing, no matter how genetically good or healthy the resultant children. And let us not forget the powerful economic interests that will surely operate in this area; with their advent, the commodification of nascent human life will be unstoppable.

### Standards, Norms and Goals

According to Genesis, God, in His creating, looked at His creatures and saw that they were *good*—intact, complete, well-working wholes, true to the spoken idea that guided their creation. What standards will guide the genetic engineers?

For the time being, one might answer, the norm of health. But even before the genetic enhancers join the party, the standard of health is being deconstructed. Are you healthy if, although you show no symptoms, you carry genes that will definitely produce Huntington's disease, or that predispose you to diabetes, breast cancer or coronary artery disease? What if you carry, say, 40 percent of the genetic markers thought to be linked to the appearance of Alzheimer's disease? And what will "healthy" and "normal" mean when we discover your genetic propensities for alcoholism, drug abuse, pederasty or violence?* The idea of health progressively becomes at

---

*Many scientists suspect that we have different inherited propensities for these and other behavioral troubles, though it is almost certain that there is no single "gene for x" that is responsible.

once both imperial and vague: medicalization of what have hitherto been mental or moral matters paradoxically brings with it the disappearance of any clear standard of health itself.

Once genetic *enhancement* comes on the scene, standards of health, wholeness or fitness will be needed more than ever, but just then is when all pretense of standards will go out the window. "Enhancement" is, of course, a euphemism for "improvement," and the idea of improvement necessarily implies a good, a better and perhaps even a best. If, however, we can no longer look to our previously unalterable human nature for a standard or norm of what is good or better, how will anyone know what constitutes an improvement? It will not do to assert that we can extrapolate from what we like about ourselves. Because memory is good, can we say how much more memory would be better? If sexual desire is good, how much more would be better? Life is good, but how much extension of the lifespan would be good for us? Only simplistic thinkers believe they can easily answer such questions.*

More modest enhancers, like more modest genetic therapists and technologists, eschew grandiose goals. They are valetudinarians, not eugenicists. They pursue not some faraway positive good, but the positive elimination of evils: diseases, pain, suffering, the likelihood of death. But let us not be deceived. Hidden in all this avoidance of evil is nothing less than the quasi-messianic goal of a painless, suffering-free and, finally, immortal existence. Only the presence of such a goal justifies the sweeping-aside of any opposition to the relentless march of medical science. Only such a goal gives trumping moral power to the principle "cure disease, relieve suffering."

"Cloning human beings is unethical and dehumanizing, you say? Never mind: it will help us treat infertility, avoid genetic disease and provide perfect materials for organ replacement." Such, indeed, was the tenor of the June 1997 report of the National Bioethics Advisory Commission on *Cloning Human Beings.* Notwithstanding its call for a temporary ban on the practice, the only moral

---

*This strikes me as the deepest problem with positive eugenics: less the threat of coercion, more the presumption of thinking we are wise enough to engineer "improvements" in the human species.

objection the commission could agree upon was that cloning "is not safe to use in humans at this time," because the technique has yet to be perfected.* Even this elite ethical body, in other words, was unable to muster any other moral argument sufficient to cause us to forgo the possible health benefits of cloning.**

The same argument will also justify creating and growing human embryos for experimentation, revising the definition of death to increase the supply of organs for transplantation, growing human body parts in the peritoneal cavities of animals, perfusing newly dead bodies as factories for useful biological substances, or reprogramming the human body and mind with genetic or neurobiological engineering. Who can sustain an objection if these practices will help us live longer and with less overt suffering?

It turns out that even the more modest biogenetic engineers, whether they know it or not, are in the immortality business, proceeding on the basis of a quasi-religious faith that all innovation is by definition progress, no matter what is sacrificed to attain it.

## The Tragedy of Success

What the enthusiasts do not see is that their utopian project will not eliminate suffering but merely shift it around. Forgetting that contentment requires that our desires do not outpace our powers, they have not noticed that the enormous medical progress of the last half-century has not left the present generation satisfied. Indeed, we are already witnessing a certain measure of public discontent as a paradoxical result of rising expectations in the health-care field: although their actual health has improved substantially in recent decades, people's *satisfaction* with their current health status has remained

---

*National Bioethics Advisory Commission, *Cloning Human Beings,* 1997, p. iii. This is, of course, not an objection to cloning itself but only to hazards tied to the technique used to produce the replicated children. For a bolder and more far-reaching assessment of cloning, see Chapter Five.

**I forbear mentioning what is rapidly becoming another trumping argument: increasing the profits of my biotech company and its shareholders, an argument often presented in more public-spirited dress: if we don't do it, other countries will, and we will lose our competitive edge in biotechnology.

the same or declined. But that is hardly the highest cost of success in the medical/humanitarian project.

As Aldous Huxley made clear in his prophetic *Brave New World,* the road chosen and driven by compassionate humaneness paved by biotechnology, if traveled to the end, leads not to human fulfillment but to human debasement. Perfected bodies are achieved at the price of flattened souls. The joys and sorrows of human attachment and achievement are replaced by factitious ecstasies that come from pills. Procreation is replaced by manufacture, family ties are absent, and people divide their time between meaningless jobs and meaningless amusements. What Tolstoy called "real life"—life in its immediacy, vividness and rootedness—has been replaced by an utterly mediated, sterile and disconnected existence. In one word: dehumanization, the inevitable result of making the essence of human nature the final object of the conquest of nature for the relief of man's estate. Like Midas, bioengineered man will be cursed to acquire precisely what he wished for, only to discover—painfully and too late—that what he wished for is not exactly what he wanted. Or, worse than Midas, he may be so dehumanized he will not even recognize that in aspiring to be perfect, he is no longer even truly human. To paraphrase Bertrand Russell, technological humanitarianism is like a warm bath that heats up so imperceptibly you don't know when to scream.

The main point here is not the rightness or wrongness of this or that imagined scenario; all this is, admittedly, highly speculative. I surely have no way of knowing whether my worst fears will be realized, but you surely have no way of knowing they will not. The point is rather the plausibility, even the wisdom, of thinking about genetic technology, like the entire technological venture (as I argued in Chapter One), under the ancient and profound idea of tragedy, in which success and failure are inseparably grown together like the concave and the convex. What I am suggesting is that genetic technology's way of approaching human life, a way spurred on by the utopian promises and perfectionist aims of modern thought and its scientific crusaders, may well turn out to be inevitable, heroic, and doomed. If this suggestion holds water, then the question regarding genetic technology is not "triumph OR tragedy," because the answer is "both together"—necessarily so.

To say that the technological approach to life, left to itself as a *way* of life, is tragic does not yet mean *our* life must inevitably be tragic. To repeat, everything depends on whether the technological disposition is allowed to proceed to its self-augmenting limits, or whether it can be restricted and brought under intellectual, spiritual, moral and political rule. But here, I regret to say, the news so far is not encouraging. For the relevant intellectual, spiritual and moral resources of our society, the legacy of civilizing traditions painfully acquired and long preserved, are taking a beating—not least because they are being called into question by the findings of modern science itself. The technologies present troublesome ethical dilemmas, but the underlying scientific notions call into question the very foundations of our ethics.

In the nineteenth and early twentieth century, the challenge came in the form of Darwinism and its seeming opposition to biblical religion, a battle initiated not so much by the scientists as by the beleaguered defenders of orthodoxy. In our own time, the challenge comes from molecular biology, behavioral genetics and evolutionary psychology, fueled by their practitioners' overconfident belief in the sufficiency of their reductionist explanations of all vital and human phenomena. Never mind "created in the image of God"; what elevated *humanistic* view of human life or human goodness is defensible against the belief, asserted by most public and prophetic voices of biology, that man is just a collection of molecules, an accident on the stage of evolution, a freakish speck of mind in a mindless universe, fundamentally no different from other living—or even nonliving—things? What chance have our treasured ideas of freedom and dignity against the reductive notion of "the selfish gene" (or, for that matter, of "genes for altruism"), the belief that DNA is the essence of life, or the teaching that all human behavior and our rich inner life are rendered intelligible only in terms of their contributions to species survival and reproductive success?

As sociologist Howard Kaye notes:

> For over forty years, we have been living in the midst of a biological and cultural revolution of which innovations such as artificial insemination with donor semen, in vitro fertilization, surrogacy, genetic manipulation, and cloning are merely technological offshoots. In both aim and impact, the end of this

revolution is a fundamental transformation in how we conceive of ourselves as human beings and how we understand the nature and purpose of human life rightly lived. Encouraged by bio-prophets like Francis Crick, Jacques Monod, E. O. Wilson and Richard Dawkins, as well as by humanists and social scientists trumpeting the essential claims of race, gender, and ethnicity, we are in the process of redefining ourselves as biological, rather than cultural and moral beings. Bombarded with white-coated claims that "Genes-R-Us," grateful for the absolution which such claims offer for our shortcomings and sins, and attracted to the promise of using efficient, technological means to fulfill our aspirations, rather than the notoriously unreliable moral or political ones, the idea that we are essentially self-replicating machines, built by the evolutionary process, designed for survival and reproduction, and run by our genes continues to gain.[7]

These transformations are, in fact, welcomed by many of our leading scientists and intellectuals. In 1997, the luminaries of the International Academy of Humanism—including biologists Crick, Dawkins and Wilson, and humanists Isaiah Berlin, W. V. Quine and Kurt Vonnegut—issued a statement in defense of cloning research in higher mammals and human beings. Their reasons were revealing:

> What moral issues would human cloning raise? Some world religions teach that human beings are fundamentally different from other mammals—that humans have been imbued by a deity with immortal souls, giving them a value that cannot be compared to that of other living things. Human nature is held to be unique and sacred. Scientific advances which pose a perceived risk of altering this "nature" are angrily opposed.... As far as the scientific enterprise can determine, [however] ... [h]uman capabilities appear to differ in degree, not in kind, from those found among the higher animals. Humanity's rich repertoire of thoughts, feelings, aspirations, and hopes seems to arise from electrochemical brain processes, not from an immaterial soul that operates in ways no instrument can discover.... Views of human nature rooted in humanity's tribal past ought not to be our primary criterion for making moral decisions about cloning.... The potential benefits of cloning may be so

immense that it would be a tragedy if ancient theological scruples should lead to a Luddite rejection of cloning.[8]

In order to justify ongoing research, these intellectuals were willing to shed not only traditional religious views but *any* view of human distinctiveness and special dignity, their own included. They failed to see that the scientific view of man they celebrated does more than insult our vanity. It undermines our self-conception as free, thoughtful and responsible beings, worthy of respect because we alone among the animals have minds and hearts that aim far higher than the mere perpetuation of our genes. It undermines, as well, the beliefs that sustain our mores, practices and institutions—including the practice of science itself. For why, on this radically reductive understanding of "the rich repertoire" of human thought, should anyone choose to accept as true the results of *these* men's "electrochemical brain processes" rather than his own? Thus do truth and error themselves, no less than freedom and dignity, become empty notions when the soul is reduced to chemicals.

The problem may lie not so much with the scientific findings themselves as with the shallow philosophy that recognizes no other truths but these and with the arrogant pronouncements of the bioprophets. For example, in a letter to the editor complaining about a review of his book *How the Mind Works,* the well-known evolutionary psychologist and popularizer Stephen Pinker rails against any appeal to the human soul:

> Unfortunately for that theory, brain science has shown that the mind is what the brain does. The supposedly immaterial soul can be bisected with a knife, altered by chemicals, turned on or off by electricity, and extinguished by a sharp blow or a lack of oxygen. Centuries ago it was unwise to ground morality on the dogma that the earth sat at the center of the universe. It is just as unwise today to ground it on dogmas about souls endowed by God.[9]

One hardly knows whether to be more impressed by the height of Pinker's arrogance or by the depth of his shallowness. But he speaks with the authority of science, and few are able and willing to dispute him on his own grounds.

There is, of course, nothing novel about reductionism, materialism and determinism of the kind displayed here; these are doctrines with which Socrates contended long ago. What is new is that, as philosophies, they seem (to many people) to be vindicated by scientific advance.* Here, in consequence, is perhaps the most pernicious result of our technological progress, more dehumanizing than any actual manipulation or technique, present or future: the erosion, perhaps the final erosion, of the idea of man as noble, dignified, precious or godlike, and its replacement with a view of man, no less than of nature, as mere raw material for manipulation and homogenization.

Hence our peculiar moral crisis. We are in turbulent seas without a landmark precisely because we adhere more and more to a view of human life that both gives us enormous power and, *at the same time,* denies every possibility of nonarbitrary standards for guiding its use. Though well equipped, we know not who we are or where we are going. We triumph over nature's unpredictability only to subject ourselves, tragically, to the still greater unpredictability of our capricious wills and our fickle opinions. Engineering the engineer as well as the engine, we race our train we know not where. That we do not recognize our predicament is itself a tribute to the depth of our infatuation with scientific progress and our naive faith in the sufficiency of our humanitarian impulses.

Does this mean that I am therefore in favor of ignorance, suffering and death? Of killing the goose of genetic technology even before she lays her golden eggs? Surely not. But unless we mobilize the courage to look foursquare at the full human meaning of our new

---

*Needless to say, I do not share these views. To the contrary, I believe that one cannot give a true account even of animals without notions of form, wholeness, awareness, appetite and goal-directed action—none of them reducible to matter-in-motion or even to DNA (see Chapter Ten). But one cannot deny the growing cultural power of scientific materialism and reductionism. The materialism of science, useful as a heuristic hypothesis, is increasingly being peddled as the one true account of human life by a new breed of bioprophets, citing as evidence the powers obtainable on the basis of just such reductive approaches to life. Many laymen, ignorant of any defensible scientific alternative to materialism, are swallowing and regurgitating these shallow soulless doctrines, because, as I say, "they *seem* to be vindicated by scientific advance." The result is likely to be serious damage to human self-understanding and the subversion of all high-minded views of the good life.

enterprise in biogenetic technology and engineering, we are doomed to become its creatures if not its slaves. Important though it is to set a moral boundary here, devise a regulation there, hoping to decrease the damage caused by this or that little rivulet, it is even more important to be sober about the true nature and meaning of the flood itself.

That our exuberant new biologists and their technological minions might be persuaded of this is, to say the least, highly unlikely. For all their ingenuity, they do not even seek the wisdom that just might yield the kind of knowledge that keeps human life human. But it is not too late for the rest of us to become aware of the dangers—not just to privacy or insurability, but to our very humanity. So aware, we might be better able to defend the increasingly beleaguered vestiges and principles of our human dignity, even as we continue to reap the considerable benefits that genetic technology will inevitably provide.

# CHAPTER FIVE

# Cloning and the Posthuman Future

Not the least of our difficulties in trying to exercise control over where biology is taking us is the fact that we do not get to decide once and for all, in an up-or-down vote, whether or not we choose for our posterity a posthuman world. The scientific discoveries and the technical powers that will take us there come to us piecemeal, one at a time and seemingly independent of one another, each often attractively introduced as a measure that will "help [us] not to be sick." But sometimes we come to a clear fork in the road where decision is possible, and where we know that our decision will make a world of difference—indeed, it will make a permanently different world. Fortunately, we stand now at the point of such a momentous choice. Events have conspired to provide us with a perfect opportunity to seize the initiative and gain some control of the biotechnical project. I refer to the prospect of human cloning, a practice absolutely central to Huxley's fictional world. Indeed, creating and manipulating life in the laboratory is the gateway to a Brave New World, not only in fiction but also in fact.

## Getting Ready for Human Cloning

The subject of cloning first came to public attention roughly thirty-five years ago, following the successful asexual production, in England, of a clutch of tadpole clones by the technique of nuclear transplantation. Largely responsible for bringing the prospect and promise of human cloning to public notice was Joshua Lederberg, a Nobel laureate geneticist and a man of large vision. Following a remarkable article in *The American Naturalist* (1966) detailing the eugenic advantages of human cloning and other forms of genetic engineering, Lederberg devoted one of his regular *Washington Post* columns on science and society to the prospect of human cloning. This, he suggested, could help us overcome the unpredictable variety that still rules human reproduction and allow us to benefit from perpetuating superior genetic endowments. These writings sparked a small public debate in which I became a participant. At the time a young researcher in molecular biology at the National Institutes of Health, I wrote a reply to the *Post,* taking strong exception to Lederberg's amoral treatment of this morally weighty subject and insisting on the urgency of confronting a series of questions and objections, culminating in the suggestion that "the programmed reproduction of man will, in fact, dehumanize him."

This newspaper exchange on cloning began a process that would soon lead me to exchange the practice of biology for a life of thinking about it and pondering its implications for how we live. In one of my first publications,[1] I discussed at length the separable ethical issues of *in vitro* fertilization and cloning—neither yet in practice—and argued that they were sequential steps down a slippery slope along which we would increasingly pay a toll in coin of our humanity and dignity for our growing technical mastery. The greatest price, I suggested, would be not the concrete harm to individuals but the erosion of support for ideas, practices and institutions long known to be central to a flourishing human life.

Much has happened in the past thirty-five years, technologically and culturally, some of it morally ambiguous. But this much is clear: we have already begun to pay that price. It has become harder, not easier, to discern the true meaning of human cloning. We have in some sense been softened up to the idea of human cloning—through movies, cartoons, jokes and intermittent commentary in the mass media, some serious, mostly lighthearted. We have become accustomed to new practices in human reproduction: not just *in vitro* fertilization, but also embryo manipulation, embryo donation, surrogate pregnancy and pre-implantation genetic diagnosis. Animal biotechnology has yielded transgenic animals and a burgeoning science of genetic engineering, easily soon to be transferable to humans.

Even more important, changes in the broader culture make it now vastly more difficult to express a common and respectful understanding of sexuality, procreation, nascent life, family and the meaning of motherhood, fatherhood and the links between the generations. Thirty years ago abortion was still largely illegal and thought to be immoral, the sexual revolution (made possible by the extramarital use of the Pill) was still in its infancy, and no one ever heard about the reproductive "rights" of single women, homosexual men and lesbians. (Never mind shameless memoirs about one's own incest!) Then I could argue, without embarrassment, that the new technologies of human reproduction—babies without sex—and their confounding of normal kin relations—who's the mother: the egg donor, the surrogate who carries and delivers, or the one who rears?—would "undermine the justification and support that biological parenthood gives to the monogamous marriage." Today, defenders of stable, monogamous marriage risk charges of giving offense to those adults who are living in "new family forms" or to those children who, even without the benefit of assisted reproduction, have acquired either three or four parents or one or none at all. Today, one must even apologize for voicing opinions that thirty years ago were almost universally regarded as the core of our culture's wisdom on these matters. In a world whose once-given natural boundaries are blurred by technological change and whose moral boundaries are seemingly up for grabs, it is much more difficult to make persuasive the still-compelling case against cloning human beings.

Indeed, perhaps the most depressing feature of the discussions that immediately followed news about Dolly, the first cloned sheep, was their ironical tone, general cynicism and moral fatigue: "An Udder Way of Making Lambs" (*Nature*), "Who Will Cash in on Breakthrough in Cloning?" (*Wall Street Journal*), "Is Cloning Baaaaaaaad?" (*Chicago Tribune*). Gone from the scene are the wise and courageous voices of Theodosius Dobzhansky (genetics), Hans Jonas (philosophy) and Paul Ramsey (theology), who thirty years ago all made powerful moral arguments against *ever* cloning a human being. We are today too jaded for such argumentation; we wouldn't be caught in public with a strong moral stance, never mind an absolutist one. We are all—or almost all—postmodernists now.

Cloning turns out to be the perfect embodiment of the ruling opinions of our new age. Thanks to the sexual revolution, we have been able to deny in practice, and increasingly in thought, the inherent procreative meaning of sexuality itself. But if sex has no intrinsic connection to generating babies, babies need have no necessary connection to sex. Thanks to feminism and the gay rights movement, we are increasingly encouraged to treat the natural heterosexual difference and its preeminence as a matter of "cultural construction." But if male and female are not normatively complementary and generatively significant, babies need not come from the union of sperm and egg. Thanks to the prominence and acceptability of divorce and out-of-wedlock births, stable monogamous marriage as the ideal home for procreation is no longer the agreed-upon cultural norm. For this new dispensation, the clone is the ideal emblem: the ultimate "single-parent child."

Although most of us profess opposition to cloning, we don't recognize or admit the degree to which cloned children would fit perfectly into the postmoral ambience in which we now live. Thanks to our belief that all children should be *wanted* children (the more high-minded principle we use to justify contraception and abortion), sooner or later only those children who fulfill our wants will be fully acceptable. Through cloning, we can work our wants and wills on the very identity of our children, exercising control as never before. Thanks to modern notions of individualism and the rate of cultural change, we see ourselves not as linked to ancestors and defined by traditions, but as projects for our own self-creation, not only as self-made men but also manmade selves; and self-cloning is simply an extension of such rootless and narcissistic self-re-creation.

Unwilling to acknowledge our debt to the past and unwilling to embrace the uncertainties and limitations of the future, we have a false relation to both: cloning personifies our desire fully to control the future while being subject to no controls ourselves. Enchanted and enslaved by the glamour of technology, we have lost our awe and wonder before the deep mysteries of nature and of life. We cheerfully take our own beginnings into our hands and, like Nietzsche's last man, we blink.

Part of the blame for our complacency lies, sadly, with the field of bioethics itself and its claim to expertise in these moral matters. Bioethics was originally founded by people who understood that the new biology touched and threatened the deepest matters of our humanity: bodily integrity, identity and individuality, lineage and kinship, freedom and self-command, eros and aspiration, and the relations and strivings of body and soul. With its capture by analytic philosophy, however, and its inevitable routinization and professionalization, the field has by and large come to content itself with abstractly analyzing moral arguments, reacting to new technological developments, and taking on emerging issues of public policy, all performed with a naive faith that the evils we fear can be avoided by compassion, regulation and a respect for autonomy. Bioethics has made some major contributions toward the protection of human subjects and in other areas where personal freedom is threatened. But with few exceptions, its practitioners have turned the big human questions into pretty thin gruel.

One reason for this is that the piecemeal formation of public policy tends to grind down large questions of morality into small questions of procedure. Many of the country's leading bioethicists have served on national commissions or state task forces and advisory boards, where, understandably, they have found utilitarianism—calculating risks and benefits, to serve the greatest good for the greatest number—to be the only ethical vocabulary acceptable to all participants in discussing issues of law, regulation and public policy. As many of these commissions have been either officially under the aegis of NIH or the Department of Health and Human Services, or else dominated by powerful advocates for scientific progress, the ethicists have for the most part been content, after some "values clarification" and wringing of hands, to pronounce their blessings upon the inevitable. Indeed, it is they, not the scientists, who are now the most articulate defenders of human cloning: when the National Bioethics Advisory Commission was preparing its report on cloning in 1997, the two witnesses who testified in favor of cloning human beings were bioethicists, eager to rebut what they regarded as the irrational concerns of those of us in opposition. If this is the teaching of *ethicists*, it is doubtful that any public commission, if similarly constituted, will free itself from the accommodationist pattern of rubber-stamping all technical innovation, in the mistaken belief that all other goods must bow down before the gods of better health and scientific advance.

While the bioethicists have dithered, the scientists have not. The work on the cloning project has proceeded rapidly. "To clone or not to clone a human being" is no longer a fanciful question. Success in cloning sheep, and also cows, mice, pigs, goats and cats, makes it perfectly clear that a fateful decision is now at hand: whether we should welcome or even tolerate the cloning of human beings. If recent newspaper reports are to be believed, reputable scientists and physicians have announced their intention to produce the first human clone in the coming year. Their efforts may already be under way.

The media, gawking and titillating as is their wont, have been softening us up for this possibility by turning the bizarre into the familiar. In the five years since the birth of Dolly the cloned sheep, the tone of discussing the prospect of human cloning has gone from "Yuck!" to "Oh?" to "Gee whiz" to "Why not?" The sentimentalizers, aided by leading bioethicists, have downplayed talk about eugenically cloning the beautiful and the brawny or the best and brightest. They have taken instead to defending clonal reproduction for humanitarian or compassionate reasons: to treat infertility in people who are said to "have no other choice," to avoid the risk of severe genetic disease, to "replace" a child who has died. For the sake of these rare benefits, they would have us countenance the entire practice of human cloning, the consequences be damned.

But we dare not be complacent about what is at issue, for the stakes are very high. Human cloning, though partly continuous with previous reproductive technologies, is also something radically new in itself and in its easily foreseeable consequences—especially when coupled with powers for genetic "enhancement" and germ-line genetic modification that may soon become available, owing to the recently completed Human Genome Project. I exaggerate somewhat, but in the direction of the truth: we are compelled to decide nothing less than whether human procreation is going to remain human, whether children are going to be made to order rather than begotten, and whether we wish to say yes in principle to the road that leads to the designer hell of *Brave New World*.

The prospect of human cloning does, in fact, provide us with a golden opportunity to make such a decision, and to exercise some control over where biology is taking us. The technology of cloning is discrete and well defined, and it requires considerable technical know-how and dexterity; we can therefore know by name many of the likely practitioners. The public demand for cloning is extremely low and most people are decidedly against it. Nothing scientifically or medically important would be lost by banning clonal reproduction; alternative and unobjectionable means are available to obtain some of the most important medical benefits claimed for (nonreproductive) human cloning. The commercial interests in human cloning are, for now, quite limited; and the nations of the world are actively seeking to prevent it. Now may be as good a chance as we will ever have to get our hands on the wheel of the runaway train now headed for a posthuman world and to steer it toward a more dignified human future.

## *The State of the Art*

What is cloning? Cloning, or asexual reproduction, is the production of individuals who are genetically identical to an already existing individual. The procedure's name is fancy—"somatic cell nuclear transfer"—but the concept is simple. Take a mature but unfertilized egg; remove or deactivate its nucleus; introduce a nucleus obtained from a specialized (somatic) cell of an adult organism. Once the egg begins to divide, transfer the little embryo to a woman's uterus to initiate a pregnancy. Since almost all the hereditary material of a cell is contained within its nucleus, the renucleated egg and the individual into which it develops are genetically identical to the organism that was the source of the transferred nucleus.

An unlimited number of genetically identical individuals—the group, as well as each of its members, is called "a clone"—could be produced by nuclear transfer. In principle, any person, male or female, newborn or adult, could be cloned, and in any quantity; and because stored cells can (if frozen) outlive their sources, one may even clone the dead. Since cloning requires no personal involvement on the part of the individual whose genetic material is used, it could easily be employed to reproduce living or deceased persons without their consent—a threat to reproductive freedom that has received relatively little attention.

Some possible misconceptions need to be avoided. Cloning is not Xeroxing: the clone of Bill Clinton, though his genetic double, would enter the world hairless and toothless and peeing in his diapers, like any other human infant. But neither is cloning just like natural twinning: the cloned twin would be identical* to an older, existing adult; it would arise not by chance but by deliberate design; and its entire genetic makeup would be preselected by its parents and/or scientists. Moreover, the success rate of cloning, at least at first, will probably not be very high. To get Dolly, the Scottish scientists transferred 277 adult nuclei into sheep eggs, implanted 29 clonal embryos, and achieved the birth of only one live lamb clone. Despite much effort, in none of the animal species in which cloning has proved successful has the success rate risen above 3 or 4 percent.

For this reason, among others, it is unlikely that, at least for now, the practice would be very popular; and there is little immediate worry of mass-scale production of multicopies. The need of repeated surgery to obtain eggs and, more crucially, of numerous borrowed (or rented) wombs for implantation will surely limit use, as will the expense. Still, for the tens of thousands of people who sustain more than three hundred assisted-reproduction clinics in the United States and already avail themselves of *in vitro* fertilization and other such techniques, cloning would be an option with virtually no added fuss. Panos Zavos, the Kentucky reproduction specialist who has announced his plans to clone a child, claims that he has already received thousands of e-mailed requests from people eager to clone, despite the known risks of failure and damaged offspring. Should commercial interests develop in "nucleus banking," as they have in sperm banking and egg harvesting; should famous athletes or other celebrities decide to market their DNA the way they now market their autographs and nearly everything else; should techniques of embryo and germ-line genetic testing and manipulation arrive as anticipated, increasing the use of laboratory assistance in order to obtain "better" babies—should all this come to pass, cloning, if it is permitted, could become more than a marginal practice simply on the basis of free reproductive choice.

---

*Perhaps not quite genetically identical. A small amount of our DNA resides not in the nucleus but in small cytoplasmic bodies called mitochondria. It is thought likely that the mitochondria of the cloned offspring will come not from the donor of the somatic cell nucleus but from the egg, though this matter has yet to be settled.

In anticipation of human cloning, apologists and proponents have already made clear some possible uses of the perfected technology, ranging from the sentimental and compassionate to the grandiose: providing a child for an infertile couple; "replacing" a loved spouse or child who is dying or has died; avoiding the risk of genetic disease; permitting reproduction for single individuals or same-sex couples; securing a genetically identical source of organs or tissues perfectly suitable for transplantation; getting a child with a genotype of one's choosing, not excluding one's own; replicating individuals of great genius, talent or beauty—having a child who really could "be like Mike"; and creating large sets of genetically identical humans suitable for research on nature versus nurture, or for special cooperative ventures in peace and war (not excluding espionage). Never mind that heredity is not quite destiny. The desire to control it through cloning has charmed more than a few prospective users, in the United States and around the world.

What are we to think about these prospects? Nothing good. Indeed, most people are repelled by nearly all aspects of human cloning: the possibility of mass production of human beings, with large groups of look-alikes, compromised in their individuality; the idea of father-son or mother-daughter "twins"; the bizarre prospect of a woman bearing and rearing a genetic copy of herself, her spouse, or even her deceased father or mother; the grotesquerie of conceiving a child as an exact "replacement" for another who has died; the utilitarian creation of embryonic duplicates of oneself, to be frozen away or created when needed to provide homologous tissues or organs for transplantation; the narcissism of those who would clone themselves, and the arrogance of others who think they know who deserves to be cloned; the Frankensteinian hubris to create a human life and increasingly to control its destiny; men playing at being God. Almost no one finds any of the suggested reasons for human cloning compelling, and almost everyone anticipates possible misuses and abuses.* And the popular belief that human cloning cannot be prevented makes the prospect all the more revolting.

---

*Over 90 percent of the American people would like to see all such human cloning banned. The figure has not wavered much in the five years since the birth of Dolly.

Revulsion is not an argument; and some of yesterday's abhorrences are today calmly accepted—not always for the better. In some crucial cases, however, repugnance is the emotional expression of deep wisdom, beyond reason's power completely to articulate it. Can anyone really give an argument fully adequate to the horror that is father-daughter incest (even with consent), or bestiality, or the mutilation of a corpse, or the eating of human flesh, or the rape or murder of another human being? Would anybody's failure to give full rational justification for his revulsion at those practices make that revulsion ethically suspect? Not at all. On the contrary, we find suspect those who think they can easily rationalize away our horror, say, by trying to explain the enormity of incest with arguments about the genetic risks of inbreeding.

I suggest that our repugnance at human cloning belongs in this category. We are repelled by the prospect of cloning human beings not because of the strangeness or the novelty of the undertaking, but because we intuit and we feel, immediately and without argument, the violation of things that we rightfully hold dear. We sense that cloning represents a profound defilement of our given nature as procreative beings, and of the social relations built on this natural ground. We also sense that cloning is a radical form of child abuse. In this age in which everything is held to be permissible so long as it is freely done, and in which our bodies are regarded as mere instruments of our autonomous rational will, revulsion may be the only voice left that speaks up to defend the central core of our humanity. Shallow are the souls that have forgotten how to shudder.

## The Context for Assessing Cloning

The goods protected by repugnance are generally overlooked by our customary ways of approaching all new biomedical technologies. The way we evaluate cloning ethically will in fact be shaped by how we characterize it descriptively, by the context into which we place it, and by the perspective from which we view it. The first task for ethics is proper description, and here is where we first begin to fail.

Typically, cloning is discussed in one or more of three familiar contexts, which one might call the technological, the liberal or the meliorist. Under the first, cloning will be seen as an extension of existing techniques for assisting reproduction and determining the genetic makeup of children. Like them, cloning is to be regarded as a neutral technique, with no inherent meaning or goodness, but subject to multiple uses, some good, some bad. The morality of cloning thus depends absolutely on the goodness or badness of the motives and intentions of the cloners. As one bioethicist defender of cloning puts it, "the ethics must be judged [only] by the way the parents nurture and rear their resulting child and whether they bestow the same love and affection on a child brought into existence by a technique of assisted reproduction as they would on a child born in the usual [!] way."

The liberal (or libertarian or liberationist) perspective sees cloning in the context of rights, freedoms and personal empowerment. Cloning is just a new option for exercising an individual's right to reproduce or to have the kind of child he or she wants. Alternatively, cloning enhances our liberation (especially women's liberation) from the confines of nature, the vagaries of chance, or the necessity of sexual mating. Indeed, it liberates women from the need for men altogether, for the process requires only eggs, nuclei and (for the time being) uteri—plus, of course, a healthy dose of our (allegedly "masculine") manipulative science that likes to do all these things to mother nature and nature's mothers. For those who hold this outlook, the only moral restraints on cloning are adequate informed consent and avoidance of bodily harm. If no one is cloned without her consent, and if the clonant is not physically damaged, the liberal conditions for licit, hence moral, conduct are met. Worries that go beyond violating the will or maiming the body are dismissed as "symbolic"—which is to say, unreal.

The meliorist perspective embraces valetudinarians and also eugenicists. The latter were more vocal in these discussions thirty years ago, but they are now generally happy to see their goals advanced under the less threatening banners of freedom and technological growth. These people see in cloning a new prospect for improving human beings—minimally, by ensuring the perpetuation of healthy individuals through avoiding the risks of genetic disease inherent in the lottery of sex, and maximally, by producing "optimum babies," preserving outstanding genetic material, and (with the help of soon-to-come techniques for precise genetic engineering) enhancing inborn human capacities on many fronts. Here the morality of cloning as a means is justified solely by the excellence of the end, that is, by the outstanding traits or individuals cloned—beauty, or brawn, or brains.

These three perspectives, all quintessentially American and all perfectly fine in their place, are sorely wanting as approaches to human procreation. It is, to say the least, grossly distorting to view the wondrous mysteries of birth, renewal and individuality, and the deep meaning of parent-child relations, largely through the lens of our reductive science and its potent technologies. Similarly, considering reproduction (and the intimate relations of family life) primarily under the politico-legal, adversarial and individualistic notion of rights can only undermine the private yet fundamentally social, cooperative and duty-laden character of childbearing, childrearing and family life and their bond to the covenant of marriage. Seeking to escape entirely from nature (in order to satisfy a natural desire or natural right to reproduce!) is self-contradictory in theory and self-alienating in practice. For we are erotic beings only because we are embodied beings, and not merely intellects and wills unfortunately imprisoned in our bodies. And though health and fitness are clearly great goods, there is something deeply disquieting in looking on our prospective children as artful products perfectible by genetic engineering, increasingly held to our willfully imposed designs, specifications and margins of tolerable error.

The technological, liberal and meliorist approaches all ignore the deeper anthropological, social and, indeed, ontological aspects and meanings of bringing forth new life. To this more fitting and profound point of view, cloning shows itself to be a major alteration—not to say violation—of our given nature as embodied, gendered and engendering beings and of the social relations built on this natural ground. Once this perspective is recognized, the ethical judgment on cloning can no longer be reduced to a matter of motives and intentions, rights and freedoms, benefits and harms, or even means and ends. It must be regarded primarily as a matter of meaning: Is cloning a fulfillment of human begetting and belonging? Or is cloning rather, as I contend, their pollution and perversion? To pollution and perversion, the fitting response can only be horror and revulsion; and conversely, generalized horror and revulsion are *prima facie* evidence of foulness and violation. The burden of moral argument must fall entirely on those who want to declare the widespread distastes of humankind to be mere timidity or superstition.

Yet repugnance need not stand naked before the bar of reason. The wisdom of our horror at human cloning can be at least partially articulated, even if this is finally one of those instances about which the heart has its reasons that reason cannot entirely know.

## The Profundity of Sex

To see cloning in its proper context, we must begin, not with laboratory technique, but with the anthropology—both natural and social—of sexual reproduction. Because this is a massive subject, only the barest outline can be suggested here, as I try to point to what is deep about the obvious.

Sexual reproduction—by which I mean the generation of new life from (exactly) two complementary elements, one female, one male, usually through coitus—is established (if that is the right term) not by human decision, culture or tradition, but by nature; it is the natural way of all mammalian reproduction. By nature, each child has two complementary biological progenitors. Each child thus stems from and unites exactly two lineages. In natural generation, moreover, the precise genetic constitution of the resulting offspring is determined by a combination of nature and chance, not by human design: each human child shares the common, natural, human genotype; each child is genetically (equally) kin to each (both) parent(s); yet each child is also genetically unique.

These biological truths about our origins foretell deep truths about our identity and about our human condition altogether. Every one of us is at once equally human, equally enmeshed in a particular familial nexus of origin, and equally individuated in our trajectory from birth to death—and, if all goes well, equally capable (despite our mortality) of participating, with a complementary other, in the very same renewal of such human possibility through procreation. Though less momentous than our common humanity, our genetic individuality is not humanly trivial. It shows forth in our distinctive appearance through which we are everywhere recognized; it is revealed in our "signature" marks of fingerprints and our self-recognizing immune system; it both symbolizes and foreshadows exactly the unique, never-to-be-repeated character of each human life.

Human societies virtually everywhere have structured child-rearing responsibilities and systems of identity and relationship on the bases of these deep natural facts of begetting. The mysterious yet ubiquitous natural "love of one's own" is everywhere culturally exploited, to make sure that children are not just produced but well cared for, and to create for everyone clear ties of meaning, belonging and obligation. But it is wrong to treat such naturally rooted social practices as mere cultural constructs (like driving on the left or the right, or like burying versus cremating the dead) that we can alter with little human cost. What would kinship be without its clear natural grounding? And what would identity be without kinship? We must resist those who have begun to refer to sexual reproduction as the "traditional method" of reproduction, and who would have us regard as merely traditional, and by implication arbitrary, what in truth is not only natural but most certainly profound.

Asexual reproduction, which produces "single-parent" offspring, is indeed a radical departure from the natural human way, confounding all normal understandings of father, mother, sibling, grandparent and the like, and all moral relations tied thereto. It becomes even more of a radical departure when the resulting offspring is a clone derived not from an embryo but from a mature adult to whom it would be an identical twin; and when the process occurs not by natural accident (as in natural twinning) but by deliberate human design and manipulation; and when the child's (or children's) genetic constitution is preselected by the parent(s) (or scientists). Accordingly, as we will see, cloning is vulnerable to three kinds of concerns and objections, related to these three points: (1) cloning threatens confusion of identity and individuality, even in small-scale practice; (2) cloning represents a giant step (though not the first one) toward transforming procreation into manufacture, that is, toward the increasing depersonalization of the process of generation and toward the "production" of human children as artifacts, products of human will and design; and (3) cloning—like other forms of eugenic engineering of the next generation—represents a form of despotism of the cloners over the cloned, and thus (even in benevolent cases) a blatant violation of the inner meaning of parent-child relations, of what it means to have a child, of what it means to say "yes" to our own demise and "replacement."

Before turning to these specific ethical objections, let me test my claim of the profundity of the natural way by taking up a challenge posed to me by a friend. Why, he wanted to know, was I making such a fuss about "the natural human way"? Why treat our sexual mode of reproduction as anything more than the accident of evolutionary history, which, like all else produced in evolutionary history, is always subject to change? What if the given natural human way of reproduction were *asexual* (rather than sexual), and we now had to deal with a new technological innovation—artificially induced sexual dimorphism and the fusing of complementary gametes— whose inventors argued cogently that sexual reproduction promised all sorts of advantages, including hybrid vigor and the creation of greatly increased individuality? Would one then be forced to defend natural *asexuality* because it was *natural?* Could one claim that it carried deep human meaning?

This is a most welcome challenge, the response to which broaches the ontological meaning of sexual reproduction and permits us to see exactly what is at stake. For it is, I submit, impossible for there to have been human life—or even higher forms of animal life—in the absence of sexuality and sexual reproduction. We find asexual reproduction only in the lowest forms of life: bacteria, algae, fungi and some lower invertebrates. Sexuality brings with it a new and enriched relationship to the world. Only sexual animals can seek and find complementary others with whom to pursue a goal that transcends their own existence. For a sexual being, the world is no longer an indifferent and largely homogeneous *otherness,* in part edible, in part dangerous. It also contains some very special and related and complementary beings, of the same kind but of opposite sex, toward whom one reaches out with special interest and intensity. In higher birds and mammals, the outward gaze keeps a lookout not only for food and predators, but also for prospective mates; the beholding of the many-splendored world is suffused with desire for union, the animal antecedent of human eros and the germ of sociality. Not by accident is the human animal both the sexiest animal—one whose females do not go into heat but are receptive throughout the estrous cycle and whose males must therefore have greater sexual appetite and energy in order to reproduce successfully—and also the most aspiring, the most social, the most open and most intelligent animal.

The soul-elevating power of sexuality is, at bottom, rooted in its strange connection to mortality, which it simultaneously accepts and tries to overcome. Asexual reproduction may be seen as a continuation of the activity of self-preservation. When one organism buds or divides to become two, the original being is (doubly) preserved, and nothing dies. In contrast, sexuality as such means perishability and serves replacement; the two that come together to generate one soon will die. Sexual desire, in human beings as in animals, thus serves an end that is partly hidden from, and finally at odds with, the self-serving individual. Whether we know it or not, when we are sexually active we are voting with our genitalia for our own demise. The salmon swimming upstream to spawn and die tell the universal story: sex is bound up with death, to which it holds a partial answer in procreation.

The salmon and the other animals evince this truth blindly. Only the human being can understand what it means. As we learn so powerfully from the story of the Garden of Eden, our humanization is coincident with sexual self-consciousness, with the recognition of our sexual nakedness and all that it implies: shame at our needy incompleteness, unruly self-division and finitude; awe before the eternal; hope in the self-transcending possibilities of children and a relationship to the divine. In the sexually self-conscious animal, sexual desire can become eros, lust can become love. Sexual desire humanly regarded is thus sublimated into erotic longing for wholeness, completion and immortality, which drives us knowingly into the embrace and its generative fruit—as well as into all the higher human possibilities of deed, speech and song.

Through children, a good common to both husband and wife, male and female achieve some genuine unification (beyond the mere sexual "union" that fails to do so). The two become one through sharing generous (not needy) love for this third being as good. Flesh of their flesh, the child is the parents' own commingled being externalized, and given a separate and persisting existence. Unification is enhanced also by their commingled work of rearing. Providing an opening to the future beyond the grave, carrying not only our seed but also our names, our ways and our hopes that they will surpass us in goodness and happiness, children are a testament to the possibility of transcendence. Gender duality and sexual desire, which first draws our love upward and outside of ourselves, finally provide for the partial overcoming of the confinement and limitation of perishable embodiment altogether.

Not by accident does Huxley's *Brave New World* begin with the overturning of sexual reproduction and its replacement by cloning. Not by accident are "birth" and "mother" regarded there as smutty notions. For to say "yes" to asexual reproduction and baby manufacture is to say "no" to all natural human relations, is to say "no" also to the deepest meaning of coupling, namely, human *erotic* longing. For human *eros* is the fruit of the peculiar conjunction of and competition between two contrary aspirations in a single living body: one, a self-regarding concern for one's own permanence and fulfillment; the other, a self-denying aspiration for something that transcends our own finite existence, and for the sake of which we spend and even give our lives. Nothing humanly fine, let alone great, will come out of a society that has crushed the source of human aspiration, the germ of which is to be found in the meaning of the sexually complementary *two* that seek unity, wholeness and holiness.

Human procreation, in sum, is not simply an activity of our rational wills. It is a more complete activity precisely because it engages us bodily, erotically and even spiritually, as well as rationally. There is wisdom in the mystery of nature that has joined the pleasure of sex, the inarticulate longing for union, the communication of the loving embrace, and the deep-seated and only partly articulate desire for children in the very activity by which we continue the chain of human existence and participate in the renewal of human possibility. Whether we know it or not—and we are already well on the way to forgetting it—the severing of procreation from sex, love and intimacy is inherently dehumanizing, no matter how good the product.

We are now ready for the more specific objections to cloning.

## *The Perversities of Cloning*

First, an important if only formal objection: Any attempt to clone a human being would constitute an unethical experiment upon the resulting child-to-be. In all the animal experiments, fewer than 3 to 4 percent of cloning attempts have succeeded. Not only are there fetal deaths and stillborn infants, but many of the so-called "successes" are in fact failures. As has only recently become clear, there is a very high incidence of major disabilities and deformities in cloned animals that attain live birth. Cloned cows often have heart and lung problems; cloned mice later develop pathological obesity; other live-born cloned animals fail to reach normal developmental milestones.

The problem, scientists suggest, may lie in the fact that an egg with a new somatic nucleus must reprogram itself in a matter of minutes or hours (whereas the nucleus of an unaltered egg has been prepared over months and years). There is thus a greatly increased likelihood of error in translating the genetic instructions, leading to developmental defects, some of which will show themselves only much later. (Note also that these induced abnormalities may also affect the stem cells that scientists hope to harvest from cloned embryos. Lousy embryos, lousy stem cells.) Nearly all scientists now agree that attempts to clone human beings carry massive risks of producing unhealthy, abnormal and malformed children. What are we to do with them? Shall we just discard the ones that fall short of expectations? Considered opinion is today nearly unanimous, even among scientists: attempts at human cloning are irresponsible and unethical. We cannot ethically even find out whether or not human cloning is feasible. (This is, of course, not an objection to cloning as such but rather to the experiments that might enable people to learn how to do it successfully.)

Second, if it were successful, cloning would create serious issues of identity and individuality. The clone may experience concerns about his distinctive identity not only because he will be, in genotype and in appearance, identical to another human being, but because he may also be twin to the person who is his "father" or his "mother"—if one can still call them that. Unaccountably, people treat as innocent the homey case of intrafamilial cloning—the cloning of husband or wife (or single mother). They forget about the unique dangers of mixing the twin relation with the parent-child relation. (For this situation, the relation of contemporaneous twins is no precedent; yet even this less problematic situation teaches us how difficult it is to wrest independence from the being for whom one has the most powerful affinity.) Virtually no parent is going to be able to treat a clone of himself or herself as one treats a child generated by the lottery of sex. No family dynamic is likely to be unaffected by the fact that the cloned child will have a special relationship to only one of his or her parents. And what will happen when the adolescent clone of Mommy becomes the spitting image of the woman with whom Daddy once fell in love? In case of divorce, will Mommy still love the clone of Daddy, even though she can no longer stand the sight of Daddy himself?

Most people talk about cloning from the point of view of adults choosing to clone. Almost nobody talks about what it would be like to be the cloned child. Surely his or her new life would constantly be scrutinized in relation to that of the older version. Even in the absence of unusual parental expectations for the clone—say, to live the same life, only without its errors—the child is likely to be ever a curiosity, ever a potential source of *déjà vu*. Unlike "normal" identical twins, a cloned individual—copied from whomever—will be saddled with a genotype that has already lived. He will not be fully a surprise to the world; people are likely always to compare his doings in life with those of his alter ego, especially if he is a clone of someone gifted or famous. True, his nurture and his circumstance will be different; genotype is not exactly destiny. But one must also expect parental efforts to shape this new life after the original—or at least to view the child with the original version always firmly in mind. For why else did they clone from the star basketball player, the mathematician, the beauty queen—or even dear old Dad—in the first place? Expectations will weigh heavily; insofar as they will be disappointed (as well they are likely to be), the question put to the cloned child will be, "How come you are *not* like the original, as we were expecting you to be?"

Third, human cloning would also represent a giant step toward the transformation of begetting into making, of procreation into manufacture (literally, making by hand), a process that has already begun with *in vitro* fertilization and genetic testing of embryos. With cloning, not only is the process in hand, but the total genetic blueprint of the cloned individual is selected and determined by the human artisans. To be sure, subsequent development is still according to natural processes, and the resulting children will be recognizably human. But we would be taking a major step into making man himself simply another one of the manmade things.

How does begetting differ from making? In natural procreation, human beings come together to give existence to another being that is formed exactly as we were, by what we are—living, hence perishable, hence aspiringly erotic, hence procreative human beings. But in clonal reproduction, and in the more advanced forms of manufacture to which it will lead, we give existence to a being not by what we are, but by what we intend and design.

Let me be clear. The problem is not the mere intervention of technique, and the point is not that "nature knows best." The problem is that any child whose being, character and capacities exist owing to human design does not stand on the same plane as its makers. As with any product of our making, no matter how excellent, the artificer stands above it, not as an equal but as a superior, transcending it by his will and creative prowess. In human cloning, scientists and prospective "parents" adopt a technocratic attitude toward human children, as their artifacts. Such an arrangement is profoundly dehumanizing, no matter how good the product.

Procreation dehumanized into manufacture is further degraded by commodification, a virtually inescapable result of allowing babymaking to proceed under the banner of commerce. Genetic and reproductive biotechnology companies are already growth industries, but they will soon go into commercial orbit now that the Human Genome Project has been completed. The sale of human eggs is already a big business, masquerading under the pretense of "donation." Newspaper advertisements on elite college campuses offer up to $50,000 for an egg "donor" tall enough to play women's basketball and with SAT scores high enough for admission to Stanford; and to nobody's surprise, at such prices there are many young coeds eager to help shoppers obtain the finest babies money can buy. (The egg-selling and womb-renting entrepreneurs shamelessly proceed on the ancient, disgusting, misogynist premise that most women will give you access to their bodies if the price is right.) Even before the capacity for human cloning is perfected, established companies will have invested in the harvesting of eggs from ovaries obtained at autopsy or through ovarian surgery, practiced embryonic genetic alteration, and initiated the stockpiling of prospective donor tissues. Through the rental of surrogate-womb services, and through the buying and selling of tissues and embryos priced according to the donor's merits, the commodification of nascent human life will be unstoppable.

Finally, the practice of human cloning by nuclear transfer—like other anticipated methods of genetically engineering the next generation—would enshrine and aggravate a profound misunderstanding of the meaning of having children and of the parent-child relationship. When a couple normally chooses to procreate, the partners are saying yes to the emergence of new life in its novelty—yes not only to having a child, but also to having whatever child this one turns out to be. In accepting our finitude, in opening ourselves to our replacement, we tacitly confess the limits of our control.

Embracing the future by procreating means precisely that we are relinquishing our grip in the very activity of taking up our own share in what we hope will be the immortality of human life and the human species. This means that our children are not our children: they are not our property, not our possessions. Neither are they supposed to live our lives for us, or to live anyone's life but their own. Their genetic distinctiveness and independence are the natural foreshadowing of the deep truth that they have their own, never-before-enacted life to live. Though sprung from a past, they take an uncharted course into the future.

Much mischief is already done by parents who try to live vicariously through their children. Children are sometimes pushed to fulfill the broken dreams of unhappy parents. Many parents already treat their children as projects, compelling them to master this or excel at that, so that the parents may bask in the reflected glory of their "product." Cloning promises to advance this perversity to a new height. For by cloning their children, such overbearing parents will have taken at the start a decisive step that—regardless of their motive for taking it—contradicts the entire meaning of the open and forward-looking nature of parent-child relations. Whereas most parents normally have hopes for their children, cloning parents will have expectations, indeed, will likely have a *plan*. The child is given a genotype that has already lived, with full expectation that this blueprint of a past life ought to be controlling the life that is to come. A wanted child now means a child who exists precisely to fulfill parental wants. Like all the more precise eugenic manipulations that will follow in its wake, cloning is thus inherently despotic, for it seeks to make one's children after one's own image (or an image of one's choosing) and their future according to one's will.

Is this hyperbolic? Consider concretely the new realities of responsibility and guilt in the households of the cloned. No longer only the sins but also the genetic choices of the parents will be visited on the children—beyond the third and fourth generation; and everyone will know who is responsible. No parent will be able to blame nature or the lottery of sex for an unhappy adolescent's big nose, dull wit, musical ineptitude, nervous disposition, or anything else that he hates about himself. Fairly or not, children will hold their cloners responsible for everything, nature as well as nurture. And parents, especially the better ones, will be limitlessly liable to guilt. Only the truly despotic souls will sleep the sleep of the innocent.

## *Answering Objections*

The defenders of cloning are not wittingly friends of despotism. Quite the contrary. They regard themselves mainly as friends of freedom: the freedom of individuals to reproduce, the freedom of scientists and inventors to discover and to devise and to foster "progress" in genetic knowledge and technique, the freedom of entrepreneurs to profit in the market. They want large-scale cloning only for animals, but they wish to preserve cloning as a human option for exercising our "right to reproduce"—our right to have children, and children with "desirable genes." As they point out, under our "right to reproduce" we already practice early forms of unnatural, artificial and extramarital reproduction, and we already practice early forms of eugenic choice. For that reason, they argue, cloning is no big deal.

We have here a perfect example of the logic of the slippery slope, and why it is slippery. Only a few years ago, arguments opposing artificial insemination donor and *in vitro* fertilization donor claimed that such innovations were only prologues: "Principles used to justify these practices will be used to justify more artificial and more eugenic practices, including cloning." "Not so," replied the defenders; "we can make the necessary distinctions." Now, without even a gesture toward making the necessary distinctions, the continuity of practice is held by itself to be justification: "Cloning is different only in small degree from what we are already doing."

The principle of reproductive freedom currently enunciated by the proponents of cloning logically embraces the ethical acceptability of sliding all the way down the slope: to producing children wholly in the laboratory from sperm to term (should it become feasible), and to producing children whose entire genetic makeup will be the product of parental eugenic planning and choice. If reproductive freedom means the right to have a child of one's own choosing by whatever means, then reproductive freedom should know and accept no limits.

Yet far from being legitimated by a "right to reproduce," the emergence of techniques of assisted reproduction and genetic engineering should compel us to reconsider the meaning and limits of such a notion. In truth, a "right to reproduce" has always been a peculiar and problematic notion. Rights generally belong to individuals, but this is a right that (before cloning) no one can exercise alone. Does the right then inhere only in couples? Only in married couples? Is it a (woman's) right to carry and deliver, or a right (of one or more parents) to nurture and rear? Is it a right to have your own "biological" child? Is it a right only to attempt reproduction, or a right also to succeed? Is it a right to acquire the baby exactly of one's choice?

The assertion of a "right to reproduce" certainly makes sense when it claims protection against state interference with procreative liberty, say, through a program of compulsory sterilization. But it surely cannot be made the basis of a tort claim against nature, to be made good by technology, should free efforts at natural procreation fail. Some insist that the right to reproduce embraces also the right against state interference with the free use of all technological means to obtain a child. Yet such a position cannot be sustained. For reasons having to do with the means employed, any community may rightfully prohibit surrogate pregnancy, polygamy, or the sale of babies to infertile couples without violating anyone's basic human "right to reproduce." When the exercise of a previously innocuous freedom now involves or impinges on troublesome practices that the original freedom never was intended to reach, the general presumption of liberty needs to be reconsidered.

We do indeed already practice negative eugenic selection, through genetic screening and prenatal diagnosis. But our practices are governed by a norm of health: We seek to prevent the birth of children who suffer from known (serious) genetic diseases. When and if gene therapy becomes possible, such diseases could then be treated, *in utero* or even before implantation—I have no ethical objection in principle to such a practice (though I have some practical worries), precisely because it serves the medical goal of healing existing individuals. But therapy, to be therapy, implies not only an existing "patient." It also implies a norm of health. In this respect, even germ-line gene "therapy," though practiced not on a human being but on egg and sperm, is less radical than cloning, which is in no way therapeutic. But once one blurs the distinction between health promotion and genetic enhancement, between "negative" and "positive" eugenics, one opens the door to all future eugenic designs. The principle "to make sure that a child will be healthy and have good chances in life" is utterly elastic, with no boundaries. Being over eight feet tall will likely produce some very good chances in life; so will having the looks of Marilyn Monroe or a genius-level intelligence.

Proponents want us to believe that there are legitimate uses of cloning that can be distinguished from illegitimate uses, yet by their own principles, no such limits can be found. (Nor could any such limits be enforced in practice: once cloning is permitted, no one ever need discover whom one is cloning and why.) Reproductive freedom, as they understand it, is governed solely by the subjective wishes of the parents-to-be. The sentimentally appealing case of the childless married couple is, on these grounds, indistinguishable from the case of an individual (married or not) who would like to clone someone famous or talented, living or dead. And the principle here endorsed justifies not only cloning but also all future artificial attempts to create (manufacture) "better" or "perfect" babies.

The "perfect baby," of course, is the project not of the infertility doctors, but of the eugenic scientists and their supporters, who, for the time being, are content to hide behind the skirts of the partisans of reproductive freedom and compassion for the infertile. For them, the paramount right is not the so-called right to reproduce, it is what the biologist Bentley Glass called, a quarter of a century ago, "the right of every child to be born with a sound physical and mental constitution, based on a sound genotype ... the inalienable right to a sound heritage." But to secure this right, and to achieve the requisite quality control over new human life, human conception and gestation will need to be brought fully into the bright light of the laboratory, beneath which the child-to-be can be fertilized, nourished, pruned, weeded, watched, inspected, prodded, pinched, cajoled, injected, tested, rated, graded, approved, stamped, wrapped, sealed and delivered. There is no other way to produce the perfect baby.

If you think that such scenarios require outside coercion or governmental tyranny, you are mistaken. Once it becomes possible, with the aid of human genomics, to produce or to select for what some regard as "better babies"—smarter, prettier, healthier, more athletic—parents will leap at the opportunity to "improve" their offspring. Indeed, not to do so will be socially regarded as a form of child neglect. Those who would ordinarily be opposed to such tinkering will be under enormous pressure to compete on behalf of their as yet unborn children—just as some now plan almost from their children's birth how to get them into Harvard. Never mind that, lacking a standard of "good" or "better," no one can really know whether any such changes will truly be improvements.

Proponents of cloning urge us to forget about the science fiction scenarios of laboratory manufacture or multiple-copy clones, and to focus only on the sympathetic cases of infertile couples exercising their reproductive rights. But why, if the single cases are so innocent, should multiplying their performance be so off-putting? (Similarly, why do others object to people's making money from that practice if the practice itself is perfectly acceptable?) The so-called science fiction cases—*Brave New World,* for instance—make vivid the meaning of what appears to us, mistakenly, to be benign. They reveal that what looks like compassionate humanitarianism is, in the end, crushing dehumanization.

## Ban the Cloning of Humans

Whether or not they share my reasons, most people, I think, share my conclusion: that human cloning is unethical in itself and dangerous in its likely consequences, which include the precedent that it will establish for designing our children. Some reach this conclusion for their own good reasons, different from my own: concerns about fairness in access to eugenic cloning; worries about the genetic effects of asexual "inbreeding"; aversion to the implicit premise of genetic determinism; objections to the embryonic and fetal wastage that must necessarily accompany the efforts; religious opposition to "man playing God." But never mind why: the overwhelming majority of our fellow Americans remain firmly opposed to cloning human beings.

For us, then, the real questions are: What should we do about it? How can we best succeed? These questions should concern everyone eager to secure deliberate human control over the powers that could redesign our humanity, even if cloning is not the issue over which they would decide to make their stand. And the answer to the first question seems pretty plain. What we should do is work to prevent human cloning by making it illegal.

We should aim for a global legal ban, if possible, and for a unilateral national ban at a minimum—and soon, before the fact is upon us. To be sure, legal bans can be violated; but we certainly curtail much mischief by outlawing incest, voluntary servitude, and the buying and selling of organs and babies. To be sure, renegade scientists may secretly undertake to violate such a law, but we can deter them by both criminal sanctions and monetary penalties, as well as by removing any incentive they have to proudly claim credit for their technological bravado.

Such a ban on clonal baby-making will not harm the progress of basic genetic science and technology. On the contrary, it will reassure the public that scientists are happy to proceed without violating the deep ethical norms and intuitions of the human community. It will also protect honorable scientists from a public backlash against the brazen misconduct of the rogues. As many scientists have publicly confessed, free and worthy science probably has much more to fear from a strong public reaction to a cloning fiasco than it does from a cloning ban, provided that the ban is judiciously crafted and vigorously enforced against those who would violate it.

What kind of a ban should we have? I have come to believe that what we need is an all-out ban on human cloning, including the creation of embryonic clones. I am convinced that all halfway measures will prove to be morally, legally and strategically flawed, and—most important—that they will not be effective in obtaining the desired result. Anyone truly serious about preventing human reproductive cloning must seek to stop the process from the beginning.

Here's why. Creating cloned human children ("reproductive cloning") necessarily begins by producing cloned human embryos. Preventing the latter would prevent the former, and prudence alone might counsel building such a "fence around the law." Yet some scientists favor embryo cloning as a way of obtaining embryos for research or as a source of cells and tissues for the possible benefit of others. (This practice they misleadingly call "therapeutic cloning" rather than the more accurate "cloning for research" or "experimental cloning," so as to obscure the fact that the clone will be "treated" only to exploitation and destruction, and that any potential future beneficiaries and any future "therapies" are at this point purely hypothetical.)

The prospect of creating new human life solely to be exploited in this way has been condemned on moral grounds by many people—including the *Washington Post,* former President Clinton, and many other supporters of a woman's right to abortion—as displaying a profound disrespect for life. Even those who are willing to scavenge so-called "spare embryos"—those products of *in vitro* fertilization made in excess of people's reproductive needs, and otherwise likely to be discarded—draw back from creating human embryos explicitly and solely for research purposes. They reject outright what they regard as the exploitation and instrumentalization of nascent human life. In addition, others who are agnostic about the moral status of the embryo see the wisdom of not needlessly offending the sensibilities of their fellow citizens who are opposed to such practices.

But even setting aside these obvious moral first impressions, a few moments of reflection show why an anti-cloning law that permitted the cloning of embryos but criminalized their transfer to produce a child would be a moral blunder. This would be a law that was not merely permissively "pro-choice" but emphatically and prescriptively "anti-life." While permitting the creation of an embryonic life, it would make it a federal offense to try to keep it alive and bring it to birth. Whatever one thinks of the moral or ontological status of the human embryo, moral sense and practical wisdom recoil from having the government of the United States on record as requiring the destruction of nascent life and, what is worse, demanding the punishment of those who would act to preserve it by (feloniously!) giving it birth.

But the problem with the approach that targets only reproductive cloning (that is, the transfer of the embryo to a woman's uterus) is not only moral but also legal and strategic. A ban only on reproductive cloning would turn out to be unenforceable. Once cloned embryos were produced and available in laboratories and assisted-reproduction centers, it would be virtually impossible to control what was done with them. Biotechnical experiments take place in laboratories, hidden from public view, and, given the rise of high-stakes commerce in biotechnology, these experiments are concealed from the competition. Stockpiles of cloned human embryos could thus be produced and bought and sold without anyone knowing it. As we have seen with *in vitro* embryos created to treat infertility, embryos produced for one reason can be used for another: today, "spare embryos" once created to begin a pregnancy are used in research, and tomorrow, clones created for research will be used to begin a pregnancy.

Assisted reproduction takes place within the privacy of the doctor-patient relationship, making outside scrutiny extremely difficult. Many infertility experts probably would obey the law, but others could and would defy it with impunity, their doings covered by the veil of secrecy that is the principle of medical confidentiality. Moreover, the transfer of embryos to begin a pregnancy is a simple procedure (especially compared with manufacturing the embryo in the first place)—simple enough that its final steps could be self-administered by the woman (if she has undergone the appropriate preparatory hormone treatments to prepare her uterus for pregnancy), who would thus absolve the doctor of blame for having "caused" the illegal transfer. (I have in mind something analogous to Kevorkian's suicide machine, which was designed to enable the patient to push the plunger and the "doctor" to evade criminal liability.)

Even should the deed become known, governmental attempts to enforce the reproductive ban would run into a swarm of moral and legal challenges, both to efforts aimed at preventing transfer to a woman and—even worse—to efforts seeking to prevent birth after transfer has occurred. A woman who wished to receive the embryo clone would no doubt seek a judicial restraining order, suing to have the law overturned in the name of a constitutionally protected interest in her own reproductive choice to clone. (The cloned child would be born before the legal proceedings were complete.) And should an "illicit clonal pregnancy" be discovered, no governmental agency would compel a woman to abort the clone, and there would be an understandable storm of protest should she be fined or jailed after she gave birth. Once the baby was born, there would even be sentimental opposition to punishing the doctor for violating the law—unless, of course, the clone turned out to be severely abnormal.

For all these reasons, the only practically effective and legally sound approach is to block human cloning at the start, at the production of the embryo clone. Such a ban can be rightly characterized not as interference with reproductive freedom, nor even as interference with scientific inquiry, but as an attempt to prevent the unhealthy, unsavory and unwelcome manufacture of and traffic in human clones.

## The Need for Prudence

Some scientists, pharmaceutical companies and bio-entrepreneurs may balk at such a comprehensive restriction. They want to get their hands on those embryos, especially for their stem cells, those pluripotent cells that can in principle be turned into any cells and any tissues in the body, potentially useful for transplantation to repair somatic damage. Embryonic stem cells need not come from cloned embryos, of course; but the scientists say that stem cells obtained from clones could be therapeutically injected into the embryo's adult "twin" without any risk of immunological rejection. It is the promise of rejection-free tissues for transplantation that so far has been the most successful public argument in favor of experimental cloning. Yet this highly touted approach strikes me as impractical at best.* Moreover, new discoveries have shown that we can probably obtain the same benefits without the need for embryo cloning.

Numerous recent studies have shown that it is possible to obtain highly potent stem cells from the bodies of children and adults—from the blood, bone marrow, brain, pancreas and fat. Beyond all expectations, these nonembryonic stem cells have been shown to have the capacity to turn into the widest variety of specialized cells and tissues. (At the same time, early human therapeutic efforts with stem cells derived from embryos have produced some horrible results, the cells going wild in their new hosts and producing other tissues

---

*One problem stems from the fact, already noted, that an embryo clone may not be entirely identical genetically to the person who donated the nucleus. A small allotment of DNA will probably come from the source of the egg, in the form of mitochondria, those small cyctoplasmic (that is, extranuclear) bodies that are responsible for energy production and have a small number of their own genes. These egg-derived genes have been shown in some animal studies to be sufficient to cause transplant rejection. Stem cells derived from cloned embryos may thus not be rejection-proof. Even were this difficulty to be surmounted, a second problem seems to rule this out as a practical clinical procedure: an enormous number of eggs will be needed in order to produce enough cloned embryos for this individualized approach. Where will these eggs come from? Because of the uncomfortable and risky hyperstimulation procedures needed, few women can be expected to donate their eggs for free; high payments for eggs will be needed. The commodification of women's reproductive tissue follows necessarily—unless, of course, animal eggs are substituted, a prospect with ethical problems of its own. There is a further practical problem, even should these others all be solved. Each therapeutic tissue, individually derived from one's own embryonic clone, would have to pass muster *individually* at the Food and Drug Administration before it could be licitly used, a daunting prospect for commercial production of useful products. All these problems make it highly unlikely that venture capital will risk backing this approach to finding successful stem cell therapies.

in addition to those in need of replacement. If an *in vitro* embryo is undetectably abnormal—as so often they are—the cells derived from it may also be abnormal.) Since cells derived from our own bodies are more easily and cheaply available than cells harvested from specially manufactured clones, we will almost surely be able to obtain from ourselves any needed homologous, transplantable cells and tissues, without the need for egg donors or cloned embryonic copies of ourselves. Moreover, the need to study the embryological development of disease processes—for which purpose scientists say they need to clone embryos from, say, diabetics or children with cystic fibrosis—can be satisfied by obtaining these nonembryonic stem cells from people with these genetic diseases. By pouring more of our resources into nonembryonic stem cell research, we can also avoid the morally and legally vexing issues in embryo research. And more to our present subject, by eschewing the cloning of embryos, we make the cloning of human beings much less likely. Given that the cloning of embryos will make cloning children more likely, and given the availability of alternative routes to the scientific and medical benefits that scientists claim may someday come from research on cloned embryos, prudence argues powerfully against permitting *any* human cloning.

Cloning need not become entangled in our old familiar political thickets. It is not an issue of pro-life versus pro-choice. It is not about death and destruction, or about a woman's right to choose. It is only and emphatically about baby design and manufacture: the opening skirmish of a long battle against eugenics and against a posthuman future. As such, it is an issue that should not divide "the left" and "the right"; and there are people across the political spectrum who are coalescing in the efforts to stop human cloning. Everyone needs to understand that, whatever we may think about the moral status of embryos, once embryonic clones are produced in laboratories the eugenic revolution will have begun. And we shall have lost our best chance to do anything about it.

As we consider the policy options, let us be clear about the urgency of our situation and the meaning of our action or inaction. Scientists and doctors whose names we know, and probably many others whose names we do not know, are today working to clone human beings. They are aware of the immediate hazards, but they are undeterred. They are prepared to screen and to destroy anything that looks abnormal. They do not care that they will not be able to detect most of the possible defects. So confident are they in their rectitude that they are willing to ignore all future consequences of the power to clone human beings. They are prepared to gamble with the well-being of any live-born clones and, if I am right, with a great deal more, all for the glory of being the first to replicate a human being. They are, in short, daring the community to defy them. In these circumstances, our silence can only mean acquiescence. To do nothing now is to accept the responsibility for the deed and for all that follows predictably in its wake.

I appreciate that a federal legislative ban on human cloning is without American precedent, at least in matters technological. Perhaps such a ban will prove ineffective. Perhaps it will eventually be shown to have been a mistake. (If so, it could later be reversed.) If enacted, however, it will have achieved one overwhelmingly important result, in addition to its contribution to thwarting cloning: it will place the burden of practical proof where it belongs. It will require the proponents to show very clearly what great social or medical good can be had only by the cloning of human beings. Surely it is only for such a compelling case, yet to be made or even imagined, that we should wish to risk this major departure—or any other major departure—in human procreation.

Americans have lived by and prospered under a rosy optimism about scientific and technological progress. The technological imperative has probably served us well, though we should admit that there is no accurate method for weighing benefits and harms. And even when we recognize the unwelcome outcomes of technological advance, we remain confident in our ability to fix all the "bad" consequences—by regulation or by means of still newer and better technologies. Yet there is very good reason for shifting the American paradigm, at least regarding those technological interventions into the human body and mind that would surely effect fundamental (and likely irreversible) changes in human nature, basic human relationships, and what it means to be a human being. Here we should not be willing to risk everything in the naive hope that should things go wrong, we can later set them right again.

Some have argued that cloning is almost certainly going to remain a marginal practice, and that we should therefore permit people to practice it. Such a view is shortsighted. Even if cloning is rarely undertaken, a society in which it is tolerated is no longer the same society—any more than is a society that permits (even small-scale) incest or cannibalism or slavery. A society that allows cloning, whether it knows it or not, has tacitly assented to the conversion of procreation into manufacture and to the treatment of children as purely the projects of our will. It has acquiesced, willy-nilly, in the eugenic redesign of future generations. The superhighway to a Brave New World lies open before this society.

But the present danger posed by human cloning is, paradoxically, also a golden opportunity. In a truly unprecedented way, we can strike a blow for the human control of the technological project, for wisdom, for prudence, for human dignity. The prospect of human cloning, so repulsive to contemplate, is the occasion for deciding whether we shall be slaves of unregulated innovation, and ultimately its artifacts, or whether we shall remain free human beings who guide our powers toward the enhancement of human dignity.

*✤Body and Soul:*
*Parts and Whole*
*in the Midst of Life*

# CHAPTER SIX

# Organs for Sale?
# Propriety, Property
# and the Price of Progress

Some time ago I was asked to review a manuscript that advocated overturning existing prohibitions on the sale of human organs in order to take advantage of market incentives to increase their supply for transplantation. Repelled by the prospect, I declined to review the article, but was later punished for my reluctance by finding it in print in a journal to which I subscribe. Reading the article made me wonder at my own attitude: what precisely was it that I found so offensive? Could it be the very idea of treating the human body as a heap of alienable spare parts? If so, is not the same idea implicit in organ *donation?* Why does payment make it seem worse? My perplexity was increased when an economically minded friend reminded me that, although we allow no commerce in organs, transplant surgeons and hospitals are making handsome profits from the organ-trading business, and even the not-for-profit transplant registries and procurement agencies glean for their employees a middleman's livelihood. Why, he asked, should everyone be making money from this business except the person whose organ makes it possible? Could it be that my real uneasiness lay with organ donation or with transplantation itself, for if not, what would be objectionable about its turning a profit?

Profit from human tissue was centrally the issue in a related development, when the California Supreme Court ruled that a patient had no property rights in cells removed from his body during surgery, cells which, following commercial genetic manipulation, became a patented cell line that now produces pharmaceutical products with a market potential estimated at several billion dollars, none of it going to the patient. Here we clearly allow commercial ownership of human tissue, but not to its original possessor. Is this fair and just? And quite apart from who reaps the profits, are we wise to allow patents for still-living human tissue? Is it really necessary, in order to encourage the beneficial exploitation of these precious resources, to allow the usual commercial and market arrangements to flourish?

With regard to organs for transplantation, voluntary donation rather than sale or routine salvage has been the norm until now, at least in the United States. The Uniform Anatomical Gift Act, passed in all fifty states some thirty years ago, altered common-law practices regarding treatment of dead bodies to allow any individual to donate all or any part of his body, the gift to take place upon his death. In 1984, Congress passed the National Organ Transplantation Act to encourage and facilitate organ donation and transplantation, by means of federal grants to organ procurement agencies and by the creation of a national procurement and matching network; this same statute prohibited and criminalized the purchase or sale of all human organs for transplant (if the transfer affects interstate commerce).

Yet in recent years, a number of commentators have been arguing for change, largely because of the shortage in organs available through donation. Some have, once again, called for a system of routine salvage of cadaveric organs, with organs regularly removed unless there is prior objection from the deceased or, after death, from his family; this is the current practice in most European countries (but not in Britain). Others, believing that it is physician diffidence or neglect that is responsible for the low yield, are experimenting with a system of required request, in which physicians are legally obliged to ask next of kin for permission to donate. Still others, wishing not to intrude upon individual rights or family feelings regarding the body of the deceased, argue instead for allowing financial incentives to induce donation, some by direct sale, others by more ingenious methods. Some years back, Lloyd Cohen proposed a futures market in organs, with individuals selling future rights to their cadaveric organs for money that will accrue to their estate if an organ is taken and used upon their death.[1] More recently, the American Medical Association has been considering proposals to provide modest contributions toward funeral expenses to families who donate organs from their newly deceased relatives.

In this business, America is not the leader of the free-market world. Elsewhere, there already exist markets in organs, indeed, in live organs. In India, for example, there is widespread and open buying and selling of kidneys, skin and even eyes from living donors—your kidney today would fetch about 25,000 rupees, or about $1200, a lifetime savings among the Indian poor. Rich people come to India from all over the world to purchase. Before Hong Kong was reunited with the People's Republic of China, the Chinese government ran ads in Hong Kong newspapers inviting people from Hong Kong to come to China for fixed-price kidney transplant surgery, with organs (from unspecified donors) and airfare included in the price. A communist country, it seems, has finally found a commodity offering it a favorable balance of trade with the capitalist West.

What are we to think of all this? For me, it is less simple than I first thought. For notwithstanding my revulsion at the idea, I am prepared to believe that offering financial incentives to prospective donors could very well increase the supply—and perhaps even the quality—of organs. I cannot deny that the dead human body has become a valuable resource which, rationally regarded, is being allowed to go to waste—in burial or cremation. Because of our scruples against sales, potential beneficiaries of transplantation are probably dying; less troubling but also true, their benefactors, actual and potential—unlike the transplant surgeons—are not permitted to reap tangible rewards for their acts of service. Finally, and most troublesome to me, I suspect that regardless of all my arguments to the contrary, I would probably make every effort and spare no expense to obtain a suitable lifesaving kidney for my own child or grandchild—if my own were unusable. And though I favor the premodern principle "One man, one liver," and am otherwise disinclined to be an organ donor, and though I can barely imagine it, I think I would readily sell one of my own kidneys, were the practice legal, if it were the only way to pay for a lifesaving operation for my children or my wife. These powerful feelings of love for one's own are certainly widely shared; though it is far from clear that they should be universalized to dictate mores or policy in this matter, they cannot be left out of any honest consideration.

The question "Organs for Sale?" is compelling and confusing also for philosophical reasons. For it joins together some of the most powerful ideas and principles that govern and enrich life in modern, liberal Western society: devotion to scientific and medical progress, for the relief of man's estate; private property, commerce and free enterprise; and the primacy of personal autonomy and choice, including freedom of contract. And yet, seen in the mirror of the present question, these principles seem to reach their natural limit or at least lose some of their momentum. For they painfully collide here with certain other notions of decency and propriety, preliberal and quasi-religious, such as the sanctity of man's bodily integrity and the respect owed to his mortal remains. Can a balance be struck? If not, which side should give ground? The stakes would seem to be high—not only in terms of lives saved or lost but also in terms of how we think about and try to live the lives we save and have.

How to proceed? Alas, this, too, poses an interesting challenge—for in whose court should one conduct the inquiry? Shall we adopt the viewpoint of the economist or the transplant facilitator or the policy analyst, each playing largely by rational rules under some version of the utilitarian ethic: find the most efficient and economical way to save lives? Or shall we adopt the viewpoint of the strict libertarian, and place the burden of proof on those who would set limits to our autonomy to buy and sell or treat our bodies in any way we wish? Or shall we adopt a moralist's position and defend the vulnerable, to argue that a great harm—say, the exploitation or degradation of even one person—cannot be overridden by providing greater goods to others, perhaps not even if the vulnerable person gives his less than fully free consent?

Further, whichever outlook we choose, from which side shall we think about restrictions on buying and selling—what the experts call "inalienability"? Do we begin by assuming markets, and force opponents to defend nonsale as the exception? Or do we begin with some conception of human decency and human flourishing, and decide how best to pursue it, electing market mechanisms only where appropriate to enhance human freedom and welfare, but remaining careful not to reduce the worth of everything to its market price? Or do we finesse such questions of principle altogether and try to muddle through, as we so often do, refining our policies on an ad hoc basis, in light of successes, costs and public pressures? Whose principles and procedures shall we accept? And on whom shall we place the burden of what sort of proof?

Because of the special nature of this topic, I will not begin with markets and not even with rational calculations of benefits and harms. Indeed, I want to step back from policy questions altogether and consider more philosophically some aspects of the *meaning* of the idea of "organs for sale." I am especially eager to understand how this idea reflects and bears on our cultural and moral attitudes and sensibilities about our own humanity and, also, to discover the light it sheds on the principles of property, free contract and medical progress. I wish, by this means, also to confront rational expertise and policy analysis with some notions outside of expertise, notions that are expressed and imbedded in our untutored repugnance at the thought of markets in human flesh. One would like to think that a proper understanding of these sentiments and notions—not readily rationalizable or measurable but not for that reason unreasonable or irrational—might make a difference to policy.

## Propriety

The nonexpert approaching the topic of organ transplantation will begin with questions of propriety, for it is through the drapings of propriety that we normally approach the human body; indeed, many of our evolved conventions of propriety—of manners and civility—are a response to the fact and problem of human embodiment. What, then, is the fit or appropriate or suitable or seemly or decent or proper way to think about and treat the human body, living and dead? This is a vast topic, yet absolutely central to our present concern; for what is permissible to do to and with the body is partly determined by what we take the human body to be and how it is related to our own being.

I have explored these questions at some length elsewhere, in an essay entitled "Thinking About the Body,"[2] from which I transplant some conclusions without the argument. Against our dominant philosophical outlooks of reductive corporealism (which knows not the soul) and person-body dualism (which deprecates the body), I advance the position of psychophysical unity, a position that regards a human being as largely, if not wholly, self-identical with his enlivened body. Looking up to the body and meditating on its upright posture and on the human arm and hand, face and mouth, and the direction of our motion (with the help of Erwin Straus's famous essay on "The Upright Posture"[3]), I argue in the following ways for the body's intrinsic dignity.

To those who know how to consider it properly, the dumb human body shows all the marks of, and creates all the conditions for, our rationality and our special way of being-in-the-world. Our bodies demonstrate, albeit silently, that we are more than just a complex version of our animal ancestors, and, conversely, more also than an enlarged brain, a consciousness somehow grafted onto or trapped within a blind mechanism that knows only survival. The body-form *as a whole* impresses on us its inner powers of thought and action. Mind and hand, gait and gaze, breath and tongue, foot and mouth—all are part of a single package, suffused with the presence of intelligence. We are *rational* (that is, *thinking*) animals, down to and up from the very tips of our toes. All equally human, we are also highly individuated and unique instances of that common humanity. This, too, the body teaches, as our faces, hands and postures display the marks of our particular incarnation of humanity, with our individual and unique identity. No wonder, then, that even a corpse still shows the marks of our common humanity as well as our distinctive version of it.

Yet this is only part of the story. We are *thinking* animals, to be sure, but we are also, simultaneously, thinking *animals*. Looking down on the body and meditating on the meaning of its nakedness (with the help of the story of man and woman in the Garden of Eden), we learn of human weakness and vulnerability, and especially of the incompleteness, insufficiency, needy dependence, perishability, self-division and lack of self-command implicit in our sexuality. While perhaps an affront to our personal dignity, these bodily marks of human abjection point also to special interpersonal relationships, as crucial to our humanity as is our rationality.

For in the navel are one's forebears, in the genitalia one's descendants. These reminders of perishability are also reminders of perpetuation; if we understand their meaning, we are even able to transform the necessary and shameful into the free and noble. The body, rightly considered, reminds us of our debt and our duties to those who have gone before. It teaches us that we are not our own source, neither in body nor in mind. Our dignity finally consists not in denying but in thoughtfully acknowledging and elevating the necessity of our embodiment, rightly regarding it as a gift to be cherished and respected. Through ceremonious treatment of mortal remains and through respectful attention to our living body and its inherent worth, we stand rightly when we stand reverently before the body, both living and dead.

This account of the meaning of the human body helps to make sense of numerous customs and taboos, some of them nearly universal. Cannibalism—the eating of human flesh, living and dead—is the preeminent defilement of the body; its humanity denied, it is treated as mere meat. Mutilation and dismemberment of corpses offend against bodily integrity. The sexual perversion of necrophilia is an offense also against the corpse and the life "it" once led. Even surgery involves overcoming repugnance at violating wholeness and taboos against submitting to self-mutilation, overridden here only in order to defend the imperiled body against still greater threats to its integrity. Voyeurism, that cannibalism of the eyes, and other offenses against sexual privacy invade another's bodily life, objectifying and publicizing what is, in truth, immediate and intimate, meaningful only within and through shared experience. Decent burial—or other ceremonial treatment—of the mortal remains of ancestors and kin pays honor to both personal identity and generational indebtedness, written, as it were, into the body itself. How these matters are carried out will vary from culture to culture, but no culture ignores them—and some are more self-consciously sensitive to these things than others.[4]

The Homeric Greeks, who took embodiment especially to heart, regarded failure to obtain proper burial as perhaps the greatest affront to human dignity. The opposite of winning great glory is not cowardice or defeat, but becoming an unburied corpse. In his invocation to the Muse at the start of the *Iliad,* Homer deplores how the wrath of Achilles not only caused strong souls of heroes to be sent to Hades, but left the heroes *themselves* to be the delicate feastings of birds and dogs. And the *Iliad* ends with the funeral of Hector, who is thus restored to his full humanity (above the animals) after

Achilles' shameful treatment of his corpse: "So they buried Hector, breaker of horses." A similarly high regard for bodily integrity comes down to us through traditional Judaism and Christianity. Indeed, the biblical tradition extends respect for bodily wholeness even to animals: while sanctioning the eating of meat, the Noahide code— widely regarded as enunciating natural rather than divine law—prohibits tearing a limb from a living animal.*

Most of our attitudes regarding invasions of the body and treatment of corpses are carried less by maxims and arguments, more by sentiments and aversions. They are transmitted inadvertently and indirectly, rarely through formal instruction. For this reason, they are held by some to be suspect, mere emotions, atavisms tied to superstitions of a bygone age. Some even argue that these aversions are based mainly on strangeness and unfamiliarity: the strange repels *because* it is unfamiliar. On this view, our squeamishness about dismemberment of corpses is akin to our horror at eating brains or mice. Time and exposure will cure us of these revulsions, especially when there are—as with organ transplantation—such enormous benefits to be won.

These views, I believe, are mistaken. To be sure, as an empirical matter, we can probably get used to many things that once repelled us—organ swapping among them. As Raskolnikov put it (and he should know), "Man gets used to everything—the beast." But I am certain that the revulsions that protect the dignity and integrity of the body are not based solely on strangeness. And they are certainly not irrational. On the contrary, they may just be—like the human body they seek to protect—the very embodiment of reason. Such was the view of Kant (whose title to rationality is second to none), writing in *The Metaphysical Principles of Virtue*:

> To deprive oneself of an integral part or organ (to mutilate oneself), for example, to *give away* or *sell* a tooth so that it can be planted in the jawbone of another person, or to submit oneself to castration in order to gain an easier livelihood as a singer, and so on, belongs to partial self-murder. But this is not

---

*This proscription is derived from the covenant with Noah, which permits the eating of meat but not blood: "Nevertheless flesh with the soul thereof which is the blood, thou shalt not eat." (Genesis 9:3-4)

the case with the amputation of a dead organ, or one on the verge of mortification and thus harmful to life. Also, it cannot be reckoned a crime against one's own person to cut off something which is, to be sure, a part, but not an organ of the body, for example, the hair, although selling one's hair for gain is not entirely free from blame.[5]

Kant, rationalist though he was, understood the rational man's duty to himself as an animal body, precisely because this special animal body was the incarnation of reason:

[T]o dispose of oneself as a mere means to some end of one's own liking is to degrade the humanity in one's person (*homo noumenon*), which, after all, was entrusted to man (*homo phaenomenon*) to preserve.[6]

Man contradicts his rational being by treating his body as a mere instrument.

Beginning with notions of propriety, rooted in the meaning of our precarious yet dignified embodiment, we start with a series of sentiments and presumptions *against* treating the human body in the ways that are required for organ transplantation, which is — once we strip away the trappings of the sterile operating rooms and their astonishing technologies — simply a noble form of cannibalism. Let me summarize these *prima facie* points of departure.

(1) Regarding *living donors,* there is a presumption against self-mutilation, even when good can come of it, a presumption, by the way, widely endorsed in the practice of medicine: Following venerable principles of medical ethics, surgeons are loath to cut into a healthy body not for its own benefit. As a result, most of them will not perform transplants using kidneys or livers from unrelated living donors.

(2) Regarding *cadaver donation,* there is a *beginning* presumption that mutilating a corpse defiles its integrity, that utilization of its parts violates its dignity, that ceremonial disposition of the total remains is the fitting way to honor and respect the life that this body once lived. Further, because of our body's inherent connection with the embodied lives of parents, spouses and children, the common law properly mandated the body of the deceased to next of kin, in order to perform last rites, to mourn together in the

presence of the remains, to say ceremonial farewell, and to mark simultaneously the connection to and the final separation from familial flesh. The deep wisdom of these sentiments and ways explains why it is a strange and indeed upsetting departure to allow the will of the deceased to determine the disposition of his remains and to direct the donation of his organs after death: for these very bodily remains are proof of the limits of his will and the fragility of his life, after which they "belong" properly to the family for the reasons and purposes just indicated. These reflections also explain why doctors—who know better than philosophers and economists the embodied nature of all personal life—are, despite their interest in organ transplantation, so reluctant to press the next of kin for permission to remove organs. This, and not fear of lawsuit, is the reason why doctors will not harvest organs without the family's consent, even in cases in which the deceased was a known, card-carrying organ donor.

(3) Regarding the *recipients of transplantation*, there is some primordial revulsion over confusion of personal identity, implicit in the thought of walking around with someone else's liver or heart. To be sure, for most recipients, life with mixed identity is vastly preferable to the alternative, and the trade is easily accepted. Also, the alien additions are tucked safely inside, hidden from sight. Yet transplantation as such—especially of vital organs—troubles the easygoing presumption of self-in-body, and ceases to do so only if one comes to accept a strict person-body dualism or adopts, against the testimony of one's own lived experience, the proposition that a person is or lives only in his brain-and/or-mind. Even the silent body speaks up to oppose transplantation, in the name of integrity, selfhood and identity: its immune system, which protects the body against all foreign intruders, naturally rejects tissues and organs transplanted from another body.

(4) Finally, regarding *privacy and publicity*, though we may celebrate the lifesaving potential of transplantation or even ordinary surgery, we are rightly repelled by the voyeurism of the media and by the ceaseless chatter about this person's donation and that person's new heart. We have good reason to deplore the coarsening of sensibilities that a generation ago thought it crude of Lyndon Johnson to show off his surgical scar, but now are quite comfortable with

television in the operating suite, requests for organ donation in the newspaper, talk-show confessions of conceiving children to donate bone marrow, and the generalized talk of spare parts and pressed flesh.

I have, I am aware, laid it on thick. But I believe it is necessary to do so. For we cannot begin in the middle, taking organ transplantation simply for granted. We must see that from the point of view of decency and seemliness and propriety, there are scruples to be overcome, and that organ transplantation must bear the burden of proof. I confess that, on balance, I believe the burden can be easily shouldered, for the saving of life is indeed a great good, acknowledged by all. Desiring the end, we will the means, and reason thus helps us overcome our revulsion—and, unfortunately, leads us to forget what this costs us in coin of shame and propriety. We are able to overcome the restraints against violating the integrity of dead bodies; less easily, but easily enough for kin, we overcome our scruple against self-mutilation in allowing and endorsing living donation—though here we remain especially sensitive to the dangers of coercion and manipulation of family ties.

How have we been able to do so? Primarily by insisting on the principle not only of voluntary consent but also of *free donation*. We have avoided the simple utilitarian calculation and not pursued the policy that would get us the most organs. We have, in short, acknowledged the weight of the nonutilitarian considerations, the concerns of propriety. Indeed, to legitimate the separation of organs from bodies, we have insisted on a principle that obscures or even, in a sense, denies the fact of ultimate separation. For in a *gift* of an organ—by its living "owner"—as with any gift, what is given is not merely the physical entity. Like any gift, a *donated* organ carries with it the donor's generous good will. It is accompanied, so to speak, by the generosity of soul of the donor. Symbolically, the "aliveness" of the organ requisite for successful transplant bespeaks also the expansive liveliness of the donor—even, or especially, after his death. Thus, organ removal, the partial alienation of self from body, turns out to be, in this curious way, a *reaffirmation* of the self's embodiment, thanks to the generous act of donation.

## Property

The most common objections to permitting the sale of body parts, especially from live donors, have to do with matters of equity, exploitation of the poor and the unemployed, and the dangers of abuse—not excluding theft and even murder to obtain valuable commodities. People deplore the degrading sale, a sale made in desperation, especially when the seller is selling something so precious as a part of his own body. Others deplore the rich man's purchase, and would group life-giving organs with other most basic goods that should not be available to the rich when the poor can't afford them (like the old Civil War practice of allowing people to purchase substitutes for themselves in the military draft). Lloyd Cohen's proposal (cited above) for a futures market was precisely intended to avoid these evils: through it he addresses only increasing the supply without embracing a market for allocation, thus avoiding special privileges for the rich; and by buying early from the living but harvesting only from the dead, he believes—I think mistakenly—that we escape the danger of exploiting the poor. (This and other half-market proposals seeking to protect the poor from exploitation would in fact cheat them out of what their organs would fetch, were the rich compelled to bid and buy in a truly open market.)

I certainly sympathize with these objections and concerns. As I read about young, healthy Indian men and women selling their kidneys to wealthy Saudis and Kuwaitis, I can only deplore the socioeconomic realities and political regimes that reduce people to such a level of desperation. And yet, at the same time, when I read the personal accounts of some who have sold, I am hard-pressed simply to condemn these individuals for electing apparently the only noncriminal way open to them to provide for a decent life for their families. As several commentators have noted, the sale of organs—like prostitution or surrogate motherhood or baby selling—creates a double bind for the poor. Proscription keeps them out of the economic mainstream, whereas permission threatens to accentuate their social alienation through the disapproval usually connected with trafficking in these matters.

Torn between sympathy and disgust, some observers would have it both ways: permit sale, but ban advertising and criminalize brokering (that is, legalize prostitutes, prosecute pimps), presumably to eliminate coercive pressure from unscrupulous middlemen. But none of these analysts, it seems to me, has faced the question squarely. For if there were nothing fundamentally wrong with trading organs in the first place, why should it bother us that some people will make their living at it? The objection in the name of exploitation and inequity, however important for determining policy, seems to betray deeper objections, unacknowledged, to the thing itself—objections of the sort I dealt with in the discussion of propriety. For it is difficult to understand why someone who sees absolutely no difficulty at all with transplantation and donation should have such trouble sanctioning sale.

True, some things freely givable ought not to be marketed because they cannot be sold; love and friendship are prime examples. So, too, are acts of generosity: it is one thing for me to offer in kindness to take the ugly duckling to the dance, but quite another for her father to pay me to do so. Yet part of the reason that love and generous deeds cannot be sold is that, strictly speaking, they cannot even be *given*—or, rather, they cannot be given *away*. One "gives" one's love to another or even one's body to one's beloved, though one does not donate it; and when friendship is "given," it is still retained by its "owner." The case with organs seems to be different. Obviously material, they clearly are freely alienable, they can be given and given away, and, therefore, they can be sold, and without diminishing the unquestioned good their transfer does for the recipient; why, then, should they not be for sale—only, of course, by their proper "owner"? Why should not the owner-donor get something for his organs? We come at last to the question of the body as property.

Even outside of law and economics, there are perhaps some commonsense reasons for regarding the body as property. For one thing, there is the curious usage of the possessive pronoun to identify my body. Often I do indeed regard my body as a tool (literally, an organ or instrument) of my soul or will. My organism is organized: for whose use?—why, for my own. My rake is mine, so is the arm with which I rake. The "my-ness" of my body also acknowledges the privacy and unsharability of my body. More important, it means also to assert possession against threats of unwelcome invasion, as in the song "My Body's Nobody's Body but Mine," which reaches for metaphysics in order to teach children to resist potential molesters. My body may or may not be mine or God's, but as between you and me, it is clearly mine.

And yet, I wonder. What kind of *property* is my body? Is it mine or is it me? Can it—or much of it—be alienated, like my other property, like my car or even my dog? And on what basis do I claim property *rights* in my body? Is it really "my own"? Have I labored to produce it? Less than did my mother, and yet it is not hers. Do I claim it on merit? Doubtful: I had it even before I could be said to be deserving. Do I hold it as a gift—whether or not there be a giver? How does one possess and use a gift? Are there limits on my right to dispose of it as I wish—especially if I do not know the answer to these questions? Can one sell—or even give away—that which is not clearly one's own?

The word "property" comes originally from the Latin adjective *proprius* (the root also of "proper"—fit or apt or suitable—and, thus, also of "propriety"), *proprius* meaning "one's own, special, particular, peculiar." Property is both that which is one's own, and also the right—indeed, the exclusive right—to its possession, use or disposal. And while there might seem to be nothing that is more "my own" than my own body, common sense finally rejects the view that my body is, strictly speaking, my property. For we do and should distinguish among that which is *me,* that which is *mine,* and that which is mine as *my property.* My body is me; my daughters are mine (and so are my opinions, deeds and speeches); my car is my property. Only the latter can clearly be alienated and sold at will.

Philosophical reflection, deepening common sense, would seem to support this view, yet not without introducing new perplexities. If we turn to John Locke, the great teacher on property, the right of property traces home in fact to the body: "Though the earth and all creatures be common to all men, yet every man has a property in his own person; this nobody has a right to but himself. The labour of his body and the work of his hands we may say are properly his."[7] The right to the fruits of one's labor seems, for Locke, to follow from the property each man has in his own person. But unlike the rights in the fruits of his labor, the rights in one's person are for Locke surely inalienable (like one's inalienable right to liberty, which also cannot be transferred to another, say, by selling oneself into slavery). The property in my own person seems to function rather to limit intrusions and claims possibly made upon me by others; it functions to exclude me—and every other human being—from the commons available to all men for appropriation and use. Thus, though the right to property stems from the my-own-ness (rather than the in-common-ness) of my body and its labor, the body itself cannot be, for Locke, property like any other. It is, like property, exclusively mine to use; but it is, unlike property, not mine to dispose of. (The philosophical and moral weakness in the very idea of property is now exposed to view: Property rights stem from the my-own-ness of my labor, which in turn is rooted in the my-own-ness of my body; but this turns out to be only relatively and politically my own.)

Yet here we are in trouble. The living body as a whole is surely not alienable, but parts of it definitely are. I may give blood, bone marrow, skin, a kidney, parts of my liver, and other organs without ceasing to be me, as the by-and-large selfsame embodied being I am. It matters not to my totality or identity if the kidney I surrendered was taken because it was diseased or because I gave it for donation. And, coming forward to my cadaver, however much it may be me rather than you, however much it will be *my* mortal remains, it will not be me; my corpse and I will have gotten divorced, and, for that reason, I can contemplate donating from it without any personal diminution. How much and what parts of the bodily me are, finally, not indispensably me, but merely mine? Do they thus become mine as property? Why or why not?

The analysis of the notion of the body as property produces only confusion—one suspects because there is confusion in the heart of the idea of property itself, as well as deep mystery in the nature of personal identity. Most of the discussion would seem to support the commonsense and common-law teaching that *there is no property in a body*—not in my own body, not in my own corpse, and surely not in the corpse of my deceased ancestor. (Regarding the latter, the common-law courts had granted to next of kin a quasi property right in the dead body, purely a custodial right for the limited purpose of burial, and one which also obliged the family to protect the person's right to a decent burial against creditors and other claimants. It was this wise teaching that was set aside by the Uniform Anatomical Gift Act.) Yet if my body is not my property, if I have no property right in my body—and here, philosophically and morally, the matter is surely dubious at best—by what right do I give parts of it away? And if it be by right of property, how can one then object—in principle—to sale?

Let us try a related but somewhat different angle. Connected to the notion of private property is the notion of free contract, the permission to transfer our entitlements at will to other private owners. Let us shift our attention from the vexed question of ownership to the principle of freedom. It was, you will recall, something like the principle of freedom—voluntary and freely given donation—that was used to justify the gift of organs, overcoming the presumption against mutilation. In contrast to certain European countries, where the dead body now becomes the property of the state, under principles of escheatage or condemnation, we have chosen to stay with individual rights. But why have we done so? Is it because we want to have the social benefits of organ transplantation without compromising respectful burial, and believe that leaving matters to individual choice is the best way to obtain these benefits? Or is the crucial fact our liberal (or even libertarian) belief in the goodness of autonomy and individual choice per se? Put another way, is it the dire need for organs that justifies opening a freedom of contract to dispose of organs, as the best—or least bad—instrument for doing so? Or is the freedom of contract paramount, and we mean to take social advantage of the right that people have to use their bodies however they wish? The difference seems to me crucial. For the principle of autonomy, separated from specific need, would liberate us for all sorts of subsequent uses of the human body, especially should they become profitable.

Our society has perceived a social need for organs. We have chosen to meet that need not by direct social decision and appropriation, but indirectly, through permitting and encouraging voluntary giving. It is, as I have argued, generosity—that is, more the "giving" than the "voluntariness"—that provides the moral ground; yet being liberals and not totalitarians, we put the legal weight on freedom, and hope that people will use it generously. As a result, it looks as if, to facilitate and to justify the practice of organ donation, we have enshrined something like the notions of property rights and free contract in the body, notions that usually include the possibility of buying and selling. This is slippery business. Once the principle of private right and autonomy is taken as the standard, it will prove difficult—if not impossible—to hold the line between donation and sale. (It will even prove impossible, philosophically, to argue against voluntary servitude, bestiality and other abominations.) Moreover, the burden of proof will fall squarely on those who want to set limits on what people may freely do with their bodies or for what purposes they may buy and sell body parts. It will, in short, be hard to prevent buying and selling human flesh not only for transplantation, but for, say, use in luxury nouvelle cuisine, once we allow markets for transplantation on libertarian grounds. We see here, in the prism of this case, the limits and, hence, the ultimate insufficiency of rights and the liberal principle.

Astute students of liberalism have long observed that our system of ordered liberties presupposes a certain kind of society—of at least minimal decency, and with strong enough familial and religious institutions to cultivate the sorts of men and women who can live civilly and responsibly with one another while enjoying their private rights. We wonder whether freedom of contract regarding the body, leading to its being bought and sold, will continue to make corrosive inroads upon the kind of people we want to be and need to be if the uses of our freedom are not to lead to our willing dehumanization. We have, over the years, moved the care for life and death from the churches to the hospitals, and the disposition of mortal remains from the clergy to the family and now to the individual himself—and perhaps, in the markets of the future, to the insurance companies or the state or enterprising brokers who will give new meaning to insider trading. No matter how many lives are saved, is this good for how we are to live?

Let us put aside questions about property and free contract, and think only about buying and selling. Never mind our rights; what would it mean to fully commercialize the human body even, say, under state monopoly? What, regardless of political system, is the moral and philosophical difference between giving an organ and selling it, or between receiving it as a gift and buying it?

The idea of commodification of human flesh repels us, quite properly I would say, because we sense that the human body especially belongs in that category of things that defy or resist commensuration—like love or friendship or life itself. To claim that these things are "priceless" is not to insist that they are of infinite worth or that one cannot calculate (albeit very roughly, and then only with the aid of very crude simplifying assumptions) how much it costs to sustain or support them. Rather, it is to claim that the bulk of their meaning and their human worth do not lend themselves to quantitative measures; for this reason, we hold them to be incommensurable, not only morally but factually.

Against this view, it can surely be argued that the entire system of market exchange rests on our arbitrary but successful attempts to commensurate the (factually) incommensurable. The genius of money is precisely that it solves by convention the problem of natural incommensurability, such as between oranges and widgets, or between manual labor and the thinking time of economists. The possibility of civilization altogether rests on this conventional means of exchange, as the ancient Greeks noted by deriving the name for money, *nomisma,* from the root *nomos,* meaning "convention"—that which has been settled by human agreement—and showing how this fundamental convention made possible commerce, leisure and the establishment of gentler views of justice.[8]

Yet the purpose of instituting such a conventional measure was to facilitate the satisfaction of *natural* human needs and the desire for well-being, and eventually, to encourage the full flowering of human possibility. Some notion of need or perceived human good provided always the latent unconventional standard behind the numismatic convention—tacitly, to be sure. And there's the rub: In due course, the standard behind money, being hidden, eventually becomes forgotten, and the counters of worth become taken for worth itself.

Truth to tell, commodification by conventional commensuration always risks the homogenization of worth, and even the homogenization of things, all under the aspect of quantity. In many transactions, we do not mind or suffer or even notice. Yet the human soul finally rebels against the principle, whenever it strikes closest to home. Consider, for example, why there is such widespread dislike of the pawnbroker. It is not only that he profits from our misfortunes and sees the shame of our having to part with heirlooms and other items said (inadequately) to have "sentimental value." It is especially because he will not and cannot appreciate their human and personal worth and pays us only their market price. How much more will we object to those who would commodify our very being?

We surpass all defensible limits of such conventional commodification when we contemplate making the convention maker—the human being—just another one of the commensurables. The end comes to be treated as merely a means. Selling our bodies, we come perilously close to selling out our souls. There is even a danger in contemplating such a prospect; for if we come to think about ourselves like pork bellies, pork bellies we will become.

We have, with some reluctance, overcome our revulsion at the exploitative manipulation of one human body to serve the life and health of another. We have managed to justify our present arrangements not only on grounds of utility or freedom but also and especially on the basis of generosity, in which the generous deed of the giver is inseparable from the organ given. To allow the commodification of these exchanges is to forget altogether the impropriety overcome in allowing donation and transplantation in the first place. And it is to turn generosity into trade, gratitude into compensation. It is to treat the most delicate of human affairs as if everything were reducible to its price.

There is a euphemism making the rounds in these discussions that makes my point. Eager to encourage more donation, but loath to condone or to speak about buying and selling organs, some have called for the practice of "rewarded gifting," in which the donor is rewarded for his generosity, not paid for his organ. Some will smile at what looks like doubletalk or hypocrisy, but even if it is hypocrisy, it is thereby a tribute paid to virtue. Rewards are given for good deeds, fees are charged for services, prices are paid merely for goods. If we must continue to practice organ transplantation, let us do so on good behavior.

Anticipating the problem we now face, Paul Ramsey thirty years ago proposed that we copy for organ donation a practice sometimes used in obtaining blood: those who freely give can, when in need, freely receive. "Families that shared in premortem giving of organs could share in freely receiving if one of them needs transplant therapy. This would be—if workable—a civilizing exchange of benefit that is not the same as commerce in organs."[9] Ramsey saw in this possibility of organized generosity a way to promote civilized community and to make virtue grow out of dire necessity. These, too, are precious "commodities," and provide an additional reason for believing that the human body and the extraordinary generosity in the gift of its parts are altogether too precious to be commodified.

## The Price of Progress

The arguments I have offered are not easy to make. I am all too well aware that they can be countered, that their appeal is largely to certain hard-to-articulate intuitions and sensibilities that I at least consider to belong intimately to the human experience of our own humanity. Precious though they might be, they do not exhaust the human picture—far from it. And perhaps, in the present case, they should give way to rational calculation, market mechanisms and even naked commodification of human flesh, all in the service of saving life at lowest cost.* Perhaps this is not the right place to draw a line or make a stand.

    Consider, then, a slightly more progressive and enterprising proposal, one anticipated by my colleague Willard Gaylin in an essay, "Harvesting the Dead," written in 1974.[10] Mindful of all the possible uses of newly dead—or perhaps not-quite-dead—bodies, kept in their borderline condition by continuous artificial respiration and assisted circulation, intact, warm, pink, recognizably you or me, but brain-dead, Gaylin imagines the multiple medically beneficial uses to which the bioemporium of such "neomorts" could be put: the neomorts could, for example, allow physicians-in-training to practice pelvic examinations and intubations without shame or fear of doing damage; serve as unharmable subjects for medical experimentation and drug testing; provide indefinite supplies of

---

*It would be worth a whole separate discussion to consider whether, in the longer view, there are not cheaper, more effective, and less indecent means to save lives, for example, through preventive measures that forestall end-stage renal disease now requiring transplantation. The definition of both need and efficiency are highly contingent, and we should beware of allowing them to be defined for us by those technologists—like transplant surgeons—wedded to present practice.

blood, marrow and skin; serve as factories to manufacture hormones and antibodies; or, eventually, be dismembered for transplantable spare parts. Since the newly dead body really is such a precious resource, why not really put it to full and limitless use?

Gaylin's scenario is not so far-fetched. Proposals to undertake precisely such body farming have been seriously discussed among medical scientists in private. The technology for maintaining neomorts is already available. Indeed, some time ago a publicly traded corporation opened a national chain of large, specialized nursing homes — or should we rather call them nurseries? — for the care and feeding solely of persons in persistent vegetative state or ventilator-dependent, irreversible coma. Roughly ten establishments each housing several hundred of such beings already exist. All that would be required to turn them into Gaylin's bioemporia would be a slight revision in the definition of death (already proposed for other reasons) — to shift from death of the whole brain to death of the cortex and the higher centers — plus the will not to let these valuable resources go to waste. Repulsive? You bet. Useful? Without doubt. Shall we go forward into this brave new world?

Forward we are going, without anyone even asking the question. In the thirty-five years since I began thinking about these matters, our society has overcome longstanding taboos and aversions to accept test-tube fertilization, commercial sperm banking, surrogate motherhood, abortion on demand, exploitation of fetal tissue, creation of human embryos solely for experimentation, patenting of living human tissue, gender-change surgery, liposuction and body shops, the widespread shuttling of human parts, assisted suicide practiced by doctors, and the deliberate generation of human beings to serve as transplant donors — not to speak about massive changes in the culture regarding shame, privacy and exposure. Perhaps more worrisome than the changes themselves is the coarsening of sensibilities and attitudes, and the irreversible effects on our imaginations and the way we come to conceive of ourselves. For there is a sad irony in our biomedical project, accurately anticipated in Aldous Huxley's *Brave New World:* We expend enormous energy and vast sums of money to preserve and prolong bodily life, but in the process our embodied life is stripped of its gravity and much of its dignity. This is, in a word, progress as tragedy.

In the transplanting of human organs, we have made a start on a road that leads imperceptibly but surely toward a destination that none of us wants to reach. A divination of this fact produced reluctance at the start. Yet the first step, overcoming reluctance, was defensible on benevolent and rational grounds: save life using organs no longer useful to their owners and otherwise lost to worms.

Now, embarked on the journey, we cannot go back. Yet we are increasingly troubled by the growing awareness that there is neither a natural nor a rational place to stop. Precedent justifies extension. So does rational calculation. Yet each new step desensitizes us to what we have lost and makes us less able to recognize the importance of what we still have to lose. We are already deeply immersed in that warm bath that heats up so imperceptibly that we don't know when to scream.

And this is perhaps the most interesting and the most tragic element of my dilemma—and it is not my dilemma alone. I don't want to encourage; yet I cannot simply condemn. I refuse to approve; yet I cannot moralize. How, in this matter of organs for sale, as in so much of modern life, is one to conduct one's thoughts if one wishes neither to be a crank nor to yield what is best in human life to rational analysis and the triumph of technique? Is poor reason impotent to do anything more than recognize and state this tragic dilemma?

❋ *Death and*
   *Immortality:*
   *Staying Human*
   *at the End of Life*

# CHAPTER SEVEN

# Is There a Right to Die?

It has been fashionable for some time now, and in many aspects of American public life, for people to demand what they want or need as a matter of rights. During the past few decades, we have heard claims of a right to health or health care, a right to education or employment, a right to privacy (embracing also a right to abort or to enjoy pornography, or to commit suicide or sodomy), a right to clean air, a right to dance naked, a right to be born, even a right not to have been born. In this atmosphere we hear much about the ultimate rights claim, a "right to die."

This claim has surfaced in connection with changing circumstances and burgeoning concerns regarding the end of life. Thanks in part to the power of medicine to preserve and prolong life, many of us are fated to end our lives in years of debility, dependence and disgrace. Thanks to the respirator and other powerful technologies that can, all by themselves, hold comatose and other severely debilitated patients on this side of the line between life and death, many who would be dead are alive only because of sustained mechanical intervention. Of the 2.2 million annual deaths in the United States, 80 percent occur in health-care facilities; in roughly 1.5 million of these cases, death is preceded by some explicit decision about stopping or not starting medical treatment. Thus, death in America is not only medically managed, but its timing is also increasingly subject to deliberate choice. It is from this background that the claims of a right to die emerge.

I do not think that the language and the approach of rights are well suited either to sound personal decision making or to sensible public policy in this very difficult and troubling matter. In most of the heartrending end-of-life situations, it is hard enough for practical wisdom to try to figure out what is morally right and humanly good, without having to contend with intransigent and absolute demands of a legal or moral right to die. And on both philosophical and legal grounds, I am inclined to believe that there can be no such thing as a *right* to die—that the notion is groundless and perhaps even logically incoherent. Even the proponents usually put "right to die" in quotation marks, acknowledging that it is at best a misnomer.

Nevertheless, we cannot simply dismiss this claim, for it raises very important and interesting practical and philosophical questions. Practically, a right to die is increasingly asserted and gaining popular strength; increasingly, we see it in print without the quotation marks. The former Euthanasia Society of America, shedding the Nazi-tainted and easily criticized "E" word, changed its name to the more politically correct Society for the Right to Die before becoming Choice in Dying. End-of-life cases coming before the courts, nearly always making their arguments in terms of rights, have gained support for some sort of "right to die." The first case to be decided by the Supreme Court, the *Cruzan* case, advanced the cause somewhat. And although in the later cases, *Glucksberg* and *Quill,* the Court unanimously refrained from finding a "right to die" in the Constitution, the reasoning of the swing opinions in these cases held open the door for a different judgment should a better case come along.

The first voter initiatives to legalize physician-assisted suicide and euthanasia in Washington and California were narrowly defeated, in part because they were badly drafted laws; yet the proponents of such practices seem to be winning the larger social battle over principle. In 1994, Oregon voters approved by referendum a Death with Dignity Act, making Oregon the first—and only—state to legalize physician-assisted suicide. According to several public opinion polls, most Americans now believe that "if life is miserable, one has the right to get out, actively and with help if necessary." Though the burden of philosophical proof for establishing new rights (especially one as bizarre as a "right to die") should always fall on the proponents, the social burden of proof has shifted to those who would oppose the voluntary choice of death through assisted suicide. Thus it has become politically necessary—and, at the same time, exceedingly difficult—to make principled arguments about why doctors must not kill, about why euthanasia is not the proper human response to human finitude, and about why there is no right to die, natural or constitutional. This is not a merely academic matter: our society's willingness and ability to protect vulnerable life against the partisans of death hang in the balance.

An examination of "right to die" is even more interesting philosophically. It reveals the dangers and limits of the liberal—that is, rights-based—political philosophy and jurisprudence to which we Americans are wedded. As the ultimate new right, grounded neither in nature nor in reason, it demonstrates the nihilistic implication of the new ("postliberal") doctrine of rights, rooted in the self-creating will. And as liberal society's response to the bittersweet victories of the medical project to conquer death, it reveals in pure form the tragic meaning of the entire modern project, both scientific and political.

The claim of a right to die is made only in Western liberal societies—not surprisingly, for only in Western liberal societies do human beings look first to the rights of individuals. Also, only here do we find the high-tech medicine capable of keeping people from dying when they might wish. Yet the claim of a right to die is also a profoundly strange claim, especially in liberal society founded on the primacy of the right to life. We Americans hold as a self-evident truth that governments exist to secure inalienable rights, first of all, the right to self-preservation; now we are being encouraged to use government to secure a putative right of self-destruction. A "right to die" is surely strange and unprecedented, and hardly innocent. Accordingly, we need to consider carefully what it could possibly mean, why it is being asserted, and whether it really exists—that is, whether it can be given a principled grounding or defense.


## A Right *to Die*

Though the major ambiguity concerns the substance of the right—namely, to die—we begin by reminding ourselves of what it means, in general, to say that someone has a right to something. I depart for now from the original notion of *natural* rights, and indeed abstract altogether from the question of the source of rights. I focus instead on our contemporary usage, for it is only in contemporary usage that this current claim of a right to die can be understood.

A right, whether legal or moral, is not identical to a need or a desire or an interest or a capacity. I may have both a need and a desire for, and also an interest in, the possessions of another, and the capacity or power to take them by force or stealth—yet I can hardly be said to have a right to them. A right, to begin with, is a species of liberty. Thomas Hobbes, the first teacher of rights, held a right to be a *blameless* liberty. Not everything we are free to do, morally or legally, do we have a right to do: I may be at liberty to wear offensive perfumes or to sass my parents or to engage in unnatural sex, but it does not follow that I have a right to do so. Even the decriminalization of a once-forbidden act does not yet establish a legal right, not even if I can give reasons for doing it. Thus, the freedom to take my life—"I have inclination, means, reasons, opportunity, and you cannot stop me, and it is not against the law"—does not suffice to establish the *right* to take my life. A true right would be at least a blameless or permitted liberty, at best a praiseworthy or even a rightful liberty, to do or not do, without anyone else's interference or opposition.

Historically, the likelihood of outside interference and opposition was in fact the necessary condition for the assertion of rights. Rights were and are, to begin with, *political* creatures, the first principles of liberal politics. The rhetoric of claiming rights, which are in principle always absolute and unconditional, performs an important function of defense, but only because the sphere of life in which they are asserted is limited. Rights are asserted to protect, by deeming them blameless or rightful, certain liberties that others are denying or threatening to curtail. Rights are claimed to defend the safety and dignity of the individual against the dominion of tyrant, king or prelate, and against those high-minded moralizers and zealous meddlers who seek to save man's soul or preserve his honor at the cost of his life and liberty.

To these more classical, negative rights against interference with our liberties, modern thought has sought to add certain so-called welfare rights, entitling us to certain opportunities or goods which, it is argued, we have a rightful claim on others—usually government—to provide. The rhetoric of welfare rights extends the power of absolute and unqualified claims beyond the goals of defense against tyranny and beyond the limited sphere of endangered liberties; for these reasons their legitimacy as rights is often questioned. Yet even these ever-expanding lists of rights are not unlimited. I cannot be said to have a right to be loved by those whom I hope will love me, or a right to become wise. There are many good things that I may rightfully possess and enjoy, but to which I have no claim if they are lacking. Most generally, then, having a right means having a *justified* claim against others that they act in a fitting manner: either that they refrain from interfering or that they deliver what is justly owed. It goes without saying that the mere assertion of a claim or demand, or the stipulation of a right, is insufficient to establish it; making a claim and actually having a rightful claim to make are not identical. In considering an alleged right to die, we must be careful to look for a *justifiable* liberty or claim, and not merely a desire, interest, power or demand.

Rights seem to entail obligations: one person's right, whether to noninterference or to some entitled good or service, necessarily implies another person's obligation. It will be important later to consider what obligations on others might be entailed by enshrining a right to die.

## A *Right to* Die

Taken literally, a right to die would denote merely a right to the inevitable; the certainty of death for all that lives is the touchstone of fated inevitability. Why claim a right to what is not only unavoidable, but even, generally speaking, regarded as an evil? Is death in danger of losing its inevitability? Are we in danger of bodily immortality? Has death, for us, become a good to be claimed rather than an evil to be shunned or conquered?

Not exactly and not yet, though these questions posed by the literal reading of "right to die" are surely germane. They hint at our growing disenchantment with the biomedical project, which seeks, in principle, to prolong life indefinitely. It is the already available means to sustain life for prolonged periods—not indefinitely, but far longer than is, in many cases, reasonable or desirable—that has made death seem less than inevitable and, when it finally does occur, appear to be a blessing.

For we now have medical "treatments" (that is, interventions) that do not treat (that is, cure or ameliorate) specific diseases, but do nothing more than keep alive by sustaining vital functions. The most notorious such device is the respirator. Others include simple yet still artificial devices for supplying food and water and the kidney dialysis machine for removing wastes. And in the future, we shall have the artificial heart. These devices, backed by aggressive institutional policies favoring their use, are capable of keeping people alive, even when comatose, often for decades. The "right to die," in today's discourse, often refers to—and certainly is meant to embrace—a right to refuse such life-sustaining medical treatment.

But the "right to die" usually embraces also something more. The ambiguity of the term blurs the difference in content and intention between the already well-established common-law right to refuse surgery or other unwanted medical treatments and hospitalization, and the newly alleged "right to die." The former permits the refusal of therapy, even a respirator, even if it means accepting an increased risk of death. The latter permits the refusal of therapy, such as renal dialysis or the feeding tube, *so that* death *will* occur. The former would seem to be more about choosing how to live while dying, the latter mainly about a choice *for death*. In this sense the claimed "right to die" is not a misnomer.

Still less is it a misnomer when we consider that some people who are claiming it demand not merely the discontinuance of treatment but positive assistance in bringing about their deaths. Here, the right to die embraces the (welfare!) right to a lethal injection or an overdose of pills administered by oneself, by one's physician, or by someone else. This "right to die" would better be called a right to assisted suicide or a right to be mercifully killed—in short, a right *to become dead*, by assistance if necessary.

This, of course, looks a lot like a claim to a right to commit suicide, which need not have any connection to the problems of dying or medical technology. Some people in fact argue that the "right to die" through euthanasia or medically assisted suicide grows not out of a right to refuse medical treatment but rather from this putative right to commit suicide (which is now decriminalized in most states). There does seem to be a world of moral difference between submitting to death (when the time has come) and killing yourself (in or out of season), between permitting to die and causing death. But the boundary becomes very fuzzy with the alleged right to refuse food and water, artificially delivered. Though few proponents of a right to die want the taint of a general defense of suicide (which, though decriminalized, remains in bad odor), they in fact presuppose its permissibility and go well beyond it. They claim not only a right to attempt suicide but a right to succeed, and this means, in practice, a *right to the deadly assistance of others.* It is thus certainly proper to understand the "right to die" in its most radical sense, namely, as a right to become or to be made dead, by whatever means.

This way of putting the matter will not sit well with those who regard the right to die less as a matter about life and death than as one of autonomy or dignity. For them, the right to die means the right to continue, despite disability, to exercise control over one's own destiny. It means, in one formulation, not the right to become dead, but the right to choose the manner, the timing and the circumstances of one's death, or the right to choose what one considers the most humane or dignified way to finish out one's life. Here the right to die means either the right to self-command or the right to death with dignity—claims that would oblige others, at a minimum, to stop interfering, but also, quite commonly, to "assist self-command" or to "provide dignity" by participating in bringing one's life to an end, according to plan. In the end, these proper and high-minded demands for autonomy and dignity turn out in most cases to embrace also a right to become dead, with assistance if necessary.

This analysis of current usage leaves us properly confused about the meaning of the term "right to die." In public discourse today, it merges all the aforementioned meanings: right to refuse treatment even if or so that death may occur; right to be killed or to become dead; right to control one's own dying; right to die with dignity; right to assistance in death. Some of this confusion inheres in the term; some of it is deliberately fostered by proponents of all these "rights," who hope thereby to gain assent to the more extreme claims by merging them with the more modest ones. Partly for this reason, however, we do well to regard "right to die" in its most radical

intention as a right to become dead, by active means and if necessary with the assistance of others. In this way we take seriously and
do justice to the novelty and boldness of the claim, a claim that
intends to go beyond both the existing common-law right to refuse
unwanted medical treatment and the so-called right to commit suicide all by oneself.* (The first right is indisputable, the second, while
debatable, I will not contest in this essay. What concerns us here are
those aspects of the "right to die" that go beyond a right to attempt
suicide and a right to refuse treatment.)

Having sought to clarify the meaning of a "right to die," we
face next the even greater confusion about who it is that allegedly

---

*In the Netherlands, we have already seen how the "right to die" has flowed down the
slippery slope to its most radical meaning and then some: from a right to refuse treatment, to a right to control one's own dying, to a right to assistance in "becoming
dead," to a right to voluntary euthanasia, to a right to be mercifully dispatched by
one's doctor should *he* decide that you are "better off dead." The descent into unau-
thorized euthanasia is confirmed by official reports from Holland, where assisted
suicide and voluntary euthanasia practiced by physicians have been encouraged for
over twenty years, under guidelines established by the medical profession. Although
the guidelines insist that choosing death must be informed and voluntary, a 1989
survey of 300 physicians disclosed that (already then) over 40 percent had performed
*non*voluntary euthanasia and over 10 percent had done so five times or more.[1]
Another survey, this one commissioned by the Dutch government, provides even more
alarming data: in 1990, besides the 2,300 cases of voluntary euthanasia and 400 cases
of physician-assisted suicide per year, there were over 1,000 cases of active *non*voluntary euthanasia performed without the patient's knowledge or consent, *including
roughly 140 cases (14 percent) in which the patients were mentally totally competent.*
(Comparable rates of nonvoluntary euthanasia for the United States would be roughly
20,000 cases per year.) In addition, there were 8,100 cases of morphine overdose with
the intent to terminate life, of which 68 percent (5,508 cases) took place without
patient knowledge or consent.[2] Responding to international criticism and concern, the
Dutch government commissioned another survey in 1995, which, the researchers
claim, shows that the practice of physician-assisted suicide and euthanasia is now well
regulated.[3] But as Dr. Herbert Hendin and his colleagues have shown by careful
scrutiny of their actual data, there remains high cause for concern. The incidence of
physician-caused death has increased since 1990 (now 4.7 percent of all deaths, up
from 3.7 percent); 59 percent of Dutch physicians, defying the requirement of notification, still do not report their death-dealing deeds; more than half feel free to suggest
euthanasia to their patients and about 25 percent admit to ending patients' lives without consent. In 1995, 948 patients were directly put to death without their consent;
another 1,896 patients died (1.4 percent of all Dutch deaths that year) as a result of
opiates given with the explicit intent to cause death (in over 80 percent of these cases,
no request for death was made by the patient).[4]

has such a right. Is it only those who are "certifiably" terminally ill and irreversibly dying with or without medical treatment? Also those who are incurably ill and severely incapacitated, although definitely not dying? Everyone, mentally competent or not? Does a senile person have a "right to die" if he is incapable of claiming it for himself? Do I need to be able to claim *and act* on such a right in order to have it, or can proxies be designated to exercise my right to die on my behalf? If the right to die is essentially an expression of my autonomy, how can anyone else exercise it for me?

Equally puzzling is the question, against whom or what is a right to die being asserted? Is it a liberty right mainly against those officious meddlers who keep me from dying—against those doctors, nurses, hospitals, right-to-life groups and district attorneys who interfere with either my ability to die (by machinery and hospitalization) or my ability to gain help in ending my life (by criminal sanctions against assisting suicide)? If it is a right to become dead, is it not also a welfare right claimed against those who do not yet assist—a right demanding also the provision of the poison that I have permission to take? (Compare the liberty right to seek an abortion with the welfare right to obtain one.) Or is it, at bottom, a demand asserted also *against nature,* which has dealt me a bad hand by keeping me alive, beyond my wishes and beneath my dignity, and alas, without terminal illness, too senile or enfeebled to make matters right?

The most radical formulations, whether in the form of "a right to become dead" or "a right to control my destiny" or "a right to dignity," are, I am convinced, the complaint of human pride against what our tyrannical tendencies lead us to experience as "cosmic injustice, directed against me." Here the ill-fated demand a right not to be ill-fated; those who want to die, but cannot, claim a right to die, which becomes, as Harvey Mansfield put it, a tort claim against nature. It thus becomes the business of the well-fated to correct nature's mistreatment of the ill-fated *by making them dead.* Thus would the same act that was only yesterday declared a crime against humanity become a mandated act, not only of compassionate charity but also of compensatory justice!

## Why Assert a Right to Die?

Before proceeding to the more challenging question of the existence and ground of a "right to die," it would be useful briefly to consider why such a right is being asserted, and by whom. Some of the reasons have already been noted in passing:

- fear of prolongation of dying due to medical intervention; hence, a right to refuse treatment or hospitalization, even if death occurs as a result;
- fear of living too long, without fatal illness to carry one off; hence, a right to assisted suicide;
- fear of the degradations of senility and dependence; hence, a right to death with dignity;
- fear of loss of control; hence, a right to choose the time and manner of one's death.

Equally important for many people is the fear of becoming a burden to others—financial, psychic, social. Few parents, however eager or willing they might be to stay alive, are pleased by the prospect that they might thereby destroy their children's and grandchildren's opportunities for happiness. Indeed, my own greatest weakening on the subject of euthanasia is precisely this: I would confess a strong temptation to remove myself from life to spare my children the anguish of years of attending my demented self and the horrible likelihood that they will come, hatefully to themselves, to resent my continued existence. Such reasons in favor of death might even lead me to think I had a *duty* to die—they do not, however, establish for me any right to become dead.*

---

*For my "generosity" to succeed, I would, of course, have to commit suicide without anyone's discovering it—that is, well before I became demented. I would not want my children to believe that I suspected them of being incapable of loving me through my inevitable decline. There is another still more powerful reason for resisting this temptation: is it not unreasonably paternalistic of me to try to order the world so as to free my children from the usual intergenerational experiences, ties, obligations and burdens? What principle of family life am I enacting and endorsing with my "altruistic suicide"? (For an excellent treatment of these matters, see Gilbert Meilaender, "I Want to Burden My Loved Ones," *First Things*, October 1991.)

But the advocates of "a right to die" are not always so generous. On the contrary, there is much dishonesty and mischief afoot. Many people have seen the advantage of using the language of rights, implying voluntary action, to shift the national attitudes regarding life and death, to prepare the way for the practice of terminating "useless" lives.

Many who argue for a right to die mean for people not merely to have it but to exercise it with dispatch, so as to decrease the mounting socioeconomic costs of caring for the irreversibly ill and dying. In fact, most of the people now agitating for a "right to die" are themselves neither ill nor dying. Children looking at parents who are not dying fast enough, hospital administrators and health economists concerned about cost cutting and waste, doctors disgusted with caring for incurables, people with eugenic or aesthetic interests who are repelled by the prospect of a society in which the young and vigorous expend enormous energies to keep alive the virtually dead—all these want to change our hard-won ethic in favor of life.

But they are either too ashamed or too shrewd to state their true intentions. Much better to hitch one's deadly purpose to the autonomy movement, trumpet a right to die, and encourage people to exercise it. These advocates understand all too well that the present American climate requires one to talk of rights if one wishes to have one's way in such moral matters. Consider the analogous use of arguments for abortion rights by organizations that hope thereby to get women—especially the poor, the unmarried and the non-white—to exercise their "right to choose," to do their supposed duty toward limiting population growth and the size of the underclass.

This is not to say that all reasons for promoting a "right to die" are suspect. Nor do I mean to suggest that it would never be right or good for someone to elect to die. But it might be dangerous folly to circumvent the grave need for prudence in these matters by substituting the confused yet absolutized principle of a "right to die," especially given the mixed motives and dangerous purposes of some of its proponents.

Truth to tell, public discourse about moral matters in the United States is much impoverished by our eagerness to transform questions of the right and the good into questions about individual rights. Partly this is a legacy of modern liberalism, the political philosophy on which the genius of the American republic mainly rests. But it is augmented by American self-assertion and individualism, increasingly so in an age in which family and other mediating institutions are in decline and the naked individual is left face to face with the bureaucratic state.

But the language of rights has gained a tremendous boost from the moral absolutism of the 1960s, with the discovery that the nonnegotiable and absolutized character of all rights claims provides the most durable battering ram against the status quo. Never mind that it fuels resentments and breeds hatreds, that it ignores the consequences to society, or that it short-circuits a political process that is more amenable to working out a balanced view of the common good. Never mind all that: go to court and demand your rights. And the courts have been all too willing to oblige, finding or inventing new rights in the process.

These sociocultural changes, having nothing to do with death and dying, surely are part of the reason we are now confronted with vociferous claims of a right to die. These changes are also part of the reason why, despite its notorious difficulties, a right to die is the leading moral concept advanced to address these most complicated and delicate human matters at the end of life. Yet the reasons for the assertion, even if suspect, do not settle the question of truth, to which, at long last, we finally turn. Let us examine whether philosophically or legally we can truly speak of a right to die.

## Is There a Right to Die?

Philosophically speaking, it makes sense to take our bearings from those great thinkers of modernity who are the originators and most thoughtful exponents of our rights-based thinking. They above all are likely to have understood the purpose, character, grounds and limits for the assertion of rights. If a newly asserted right, such as the right to die, cannot be established on the natural or rational ground for rights offered by these thinkers, the burden of proof must fall on the proponents of novel rights, to provide a new yet equally solid ground in support of their novel claims.

If we start at the beginning, with the great philosophical teachers of natural rights, the very notion of a right to die is nonsensical.

As we learn from Hobbes and from John Locke, all the rights of man, given by nature, presuppose our self-interested attachment to our own lives. All natural rights trace home to the primary right to life, or, better, the right to self-preservation—itself rooted in the powerful, self-loving impulses and passions that seek our own continuance, and asserted first against deadly oppressive polities or against those who might insist that morality requires me to turn the other cheek when my life is threatened. Harvey Mansfield summarizes the classical position elegantly:

> Rights are given to men by nature, but they are needed because men are also subject to nature's improvidence. Since life is in danger, men's equal rights would be to life, to the liberty that protects life, and to the pursuit of the happiness with which life, or a tenuous life, is occupied.
>
> In practice, the pursuit of happiness will be the pursuit of property, for even though property is less valuable than life or liberty, it serves as guard for them. Quite apart from the pleasures of being rich, having secure property shows that one has liberty secure from invasion either by the government or by others; and secure liberty is the best sign of a secure life.[5]

Because death, my extinction, is the evil whose avoidance is the condition of the possibility of any and all of my goods, my right to secure my life against death—that is, my rightful liberty to self-preservative conduct—is the bedrock of all other rights and of all politically relevant morality. Even Hans Jonas, writing to defend "the right to die," acknowledges that it stands alone, and concedes that "every other right ever argued, claimed, granted, or denied can be viewed as an extension of this primary right [to life], since every particular right concerns the exercise of some faculty of life, the access to some necessity of life, the satisfaction of some aspiration of life."[6] It is obvious that one cannot found on this rock any "right to die" or "right to become dead." Life loves to live, and needs all the help it can get.

This is not to say that these early modern thinkers were unaware that men might tire of life or come to find existence burdensome. But the decline in the will to live did not for them drive out or nullify the right to life, much less lead to a trumping new right, a right to die. For the right to life is a matter of nature, not will. Locke addresses and rejects a natural right to suicide in his discussion of the state of nature:

> But though this be a state of liberty, yet it is not a state of license; though man in that state has an uncontrollable liberty to dispose of his person or possessions, yet he has not liberty to destroy himself, or so much as any creature in his possession, but where some nobler use than its bare preservation calls for it. The state of nature has a law of nature to govern it, which obliges everyone; and reason, which is that law, teaches all mankind who will but consult it, that, being all equal and independent, no one ought to harm another in his life, health, liberty, or possessions.[7]

Admittedly, the argument here turns explicitly theological—we are said to be our wise Maker's property. But the argument against a man's willful "quitting of his station" seems, for Locke, to be a corollary of the natural inclination and right of self-preservation.

Some try to argue, wrongly in my view, that Locke's teaching on property rests on a principle of self-ownership, which can then be used to justify self-destruction: since I own my body and my life, I may do with them as I please. As this argument has much currency, it is worth examining it in greater detail. Locke does, indeed, say something that seems at first glance to suggest self-ownership: "Though the earth and all inferior creatures be common to all men, *yet every man has a property in his own person;* this nobody has a right to but himself. The labor of his body and the work of his hands we may say are properly his."[8]

But the context defines and constricts the claim. Unlike the property rights in the fruits of his labor, the property a man has in his own person is inalienable: a man cannot transfer title to himself by selling himself into slavery. The "property in his own person" is less a metaphysical statement declaring self-ownership than a political statement denying ownership by another. This right moves each and every human being from the commons available to all human beings for appropriation and use. My body and my life are my property *only in the limited sense* that they are *not yours*. They are different from my alienable property—my house, my car, my shoes.

My body and my life, while mine to use, are not mine to dispose of. In the deepest sense, my body is nobody's body, not even mine.*

Even if one continues, against reason, to hold to strict self-ownership and self-disposability, there is one further argument, one that is decisive. Self-ownership might enable one at most to justify *attempting* suicide; it cannot justify a right to succeed or, more important, a right to the assistance of others. The designated potential assistant-in-death has neither a natural duty nor a natural right to become an actual assistant-in-death, and the liberal state, instituted above all to protect life, can never countenance such a right to kill, even on request. A right to become dead or to be made dead cannot be sustained on classical liberal grounds.

Later thinkers in the liberal tradition, including those who prized freedom above preservation, also make no room for a "right to die." Jean-Jacques Rousseau's complaints about the ills of civil society centered especially and most powerfully on the threats to life and limb from a social order whose main purpose should have been to protect them.[9] And Immanuel Kant, for whom rights are founded not in nature but in reason, holds that the self-willed act of self-destruction is simply self-contradictory.

> It seems absurd that a man can injure himself (*volenti non fit injuria* [Injury cannot happen to one who is willing]). The Stoic therefore considered it a prerogative of his personality as a wise man to walk out of his life with an undisturbed mind whenever he liked (as out of a smoke-filled room), not because he was afflicted by actual or anticipated ills, but simply because he could make use of nothing more in this life. And yet this very courage, this strength of mind—of not fearing death and of knowing of something which man can prize more highly than

---

*Later, in discussing the extent of legislative power, Locke denies to the legislative, though it be the supreme power in every commonwealth, arbitrary power over the individual, and, in particular, power to destroy his life. "For nobody can transfer to another more power than he has in himself; and nobody has an absolute arbitrary power over himself, or over any other to destroy his own life, or take away the life or property of another." (*Second Treatise,* Chapter XI, "Of the Extent of the Legislative Power," par. 135) Because the state's power derives from the people's, the person's lack of arbitrary power over himself is the ground for restricting the state's power to kill him.

his life—ought to have been an ever so much greater motive for him not to destroy himself, a being having such authoritative superiority over the strongest sensible incentives; consequently, it ought to have been a motive for him not to deprive himself of life.

Man cannot deprive himself of his personhood so long as one speaks of duties, thus so long as he lives. That man ought to have the authorization to withdraw himself from all obligation, i.e. to be free to act as if no authorization at all were required for this withdrawal, involves a contradiction. To destroy the subject of morality in his own person is tantamount to obliterating from the world, as far as he can, the very existence of morality itself; but morality is, nevertheless, an end in itself. Accordingly, to dispose of oneself as a mere means to some end of one's own liking is to degrade the humanity in one's person (*homo noumenon*), which, after all, was entrusted to man (*homo phaenomenon*) to preserve.[10]

It is a heavy irony that it should be autonomy, the moral notion the world owes mainly to Kant, that is now invoked as the justifying ground of a right to die. For Kant, autonomy, which literally means "self-legislation," requires acting in accordance with one's true self—that is, with one's rational will determined by a universalizable, that is, rational maxim. Being autonomous means not being a slave to instinct, impulse or whim, but rather doing as one ought, as a rational being. But "autonomy" has now come to mean "doing as you please," compatible no less with self-indulgence than with self-control. Herewith, one sees clearly the triumph of the Nietzschean self, who finds reason just as enslaving as blind instinct and who finds his true "self" rather in unconditioned acts of pure creative will.

Yet even in its willful modern meaning, "autonomy" cannot ground a right to die. First, one cannot establish on this basis a right to have *someone else's* assistance in committing suicide—a right, by the way, that would impose an obligation on someone else and thereby restrict *his* autonomy. Second, even if my choice for death were "reasonable" and my chosen assistant freely willing, my autonomy cannot ground *his right* to kill me, and hence, it cannot ground my right to become dead. Third, a liberty right to an assisted death (that is, a right against interference) can at most approve assisted suicide or euthanasia for the mentally competent and alert—a restriction that would prohibit effecting the deaths of the mentally incompetent or comatose patients who have not left explicit instructions regarding their treatment. It is, by the way, a long philosophical question whether all such instructions must be obeyed, for the person who gave them long ago may no longer be "the same person" when they become relevant. Can my 63-year-old self truly prescribe today the best interests for my 75-year-old and senile self?

In contrast to arguments presented in recent court cases, it is self-contradictory to assert that a proxy not chosen by the patient can exercise the patient's rights of autonomy. Can a citizen have a right to vote that would be irrevocably exercised "on his behalf," and in the name of his autonomy, by the government?* Finally, if autonomy and dignity lie in the free exercise of will and choice, it is at least paradoxical to say that our autonomy licenses an act that puts our autonomy permanently out of business.

It is precisely this paradox that appeals to the Nietzschean creative self, the bearer of so many of this century's "new rights." As Mansfield brilliantly shows, the creative ones are not bound by normality or good sense:

> Creative beings are open-ended. They are open-ended in fact and not merely in their formal potentialities. Such beings do not have interests; for who can say what is in the interest of a being that is becoming something unknown? Thus the society of new rights is characterized by a loss of predictability and normality: no one knows what to expect, even from his closest companions.[11]

The most authentic, self-creative self revels in the unpredictable, the extreme, the perverse. He does not even flinch before self-contradiction; indeed, he can display the triumph of his will most especially in self-negation. And though it may revolt us, who are we

---

*The attempt to ground a right to die in the "right to privacy" fails for the same reasons. A right to make independent judgments regarding one's body in one's private sphere, free of governmental interference, cannot be the basis of the right of someone else, appointed by or protected by government, to put an end to one's bodily life.

to deny him this form of self-expression? Supremely tolerant of the rights of others to their own eccentricities, we avert our glance and turn the other moral cheek. Here at last is the only possible philo-sophical ground for a right to die: arbitrary will, backed by moral relativism. Which is to say, no ground at all.

## Is There a Legal Right to Die?

Such foreign philosophic doctrines, prominent among the elite, are slowly working their relativistic way through the broader culture. But in America, rights are still largely defined by law, most promi-nently constitutional law. Turning, then, from political and moral philosophy to American constitutional law, we should be surprised to discover any constitutional basis for a legal right to die, given that the framers understood rights and the role of government more or less as did Locke. Perusal of the Constitution finds absolutely no textual basis or support for such a right.

But the notorious Due Process Clause of the Fourteenth Amend-ment, under the ruling but still oxymoronic "substantive due process" interpretation, has provided such a possible peg, as it has for so many other new rights, notwithstanding the fact that the majority of states at the time the Fourteenth Amendment was ratified had laws that prohibited assisting suicide. The Supreme Court has now twice issued opinions in "right to die" cases. In 1990 the Court, by a five-to-four vote in *Cruzan by Cruzan v. Director, Missouri Depart-ment of Health,* first explored the Fourteenth Amendment in con-nection with such a right, nominally ruling in favor of the state and against the "right to die."[12] In 1997 the Court again spoke to the issue, in two companion cases, *Washington v. Glucksberg* and *Vacco v. Quill,* once more ruling in favor of the state, this time unani-mously.[13] A careful examination of these cases, especially the latter pair, reveals little enthusiasm for the creation of a constitutional right to die, but also less than majority support for closing the door on the possibility. Indeed, the most remarkable feature of these two "victories" for the state against claims of a "right to die" is the Court's failure to reject the claimed "right to die" in categorical terms. In the end, the present Court seems willing to let the legislative process wrestle with the issue, but it also seems unwilling to tie the hands of its successors, leaving open the possibility that a "right to die" majority opinion might still one day be written.

The *Cruzan* decision opened the door to a constitutional right to die. The parents of Nancy Cruzan, a comatose young woman living for seven years in a persistent vegetative state, petitioned to remove the gastrostomy feeding and hydration tube in order that Nancy be allowed to die. The trial court found for the parents, but the Missouri Supreme Court reversed; when the Cruzans appealed, the United States Supreme Court took the case to consider "whether Cruzan has a right under the United States Constitution which would require the hospital to withdraw life-sustaining treatment from her under the circumstances."

At first glance, the Court's decision in *Cruzan* disappointed proponents of a right to die because it upheld the decision of the Missouri Supreme Court: it held that Missouri's interest in safeguarding life allowed it to demand clear and convincing evidence that the incompetent person truly wished to withdraw from treatment, evidence that in Nancy's case was lacking. Nevertheless, the reasoning of the majority decision was widely interpreted as conceding such a right to die for a competent person—a misinterpretation, to be sure, but not without some ground.

Chief Justice William Rehnquist, writing for the majority, scrupulously avoided any mention of a "right to die," and he wisely eschewed taking up the question under the so-called right of privacy. Instead, following precedent in Fourteenth Amendment jurisprudence and relying on the doctrine that informed consent is required for medical invasion of the body, he reasoned that "the principle that a competent person has a constitutionally protected liberty interest in *refusing unwanted medical treatment* may be inferred from our previous decisions." (A "liberty interest" is a technical term denoting a liberty less firmly protected by the Due Process Clause than a "fundamental right"; generally speaking, restrictions on the latter may be justified only by the Court's most demanding "compelling state interest" test, but restraints on the former may be upheld if they pass the ill-defined but less exacting "no undue burden" test.) If a competent person is sick, our legal tradition recognizes that he must *want* to be made well; the state cannot force him to have an operation or take his medication.

The Cruzan case might have tested whether that general principle can be stretched to its outer limit. Does the protected liberty interest to refuse medical treatment embrace also refusing *life-sustaining* food and water? On this crucial question, Rehnquist waffled skillfully:

> Petitioners insist that under the general holdings of our cases, the forced administration of life-sustaining medical treatment, and even of artificially-delivered food and water essential to life, would implicate a competent person's liberty interest. Although we think the logic of the cases discussed above would embrace such a liberty interest, the dramatic consequences involved in refusal of such treatment [namely death] would inform the inquiry whether the deprivation of that interest is constitutionally permissible. *But for purposes of this case, we assume that the United States Constitution would grant a competent person a constitutionally protected right to refuse life-saving hydration and nutrition.* [p. 279; emphasis added.]

The emphasized portion of this passage in Rehnquist's opinion was seized upon by the media as expressing support for a competent patient's liberty interest in refusing lifesaving treatment. Little noticed was the sentence that precedes it, which rather conspicuously raises the opposite possibility. Even though the common-law liberty to refuse medical treatment is well established, the Court still might choose not to recognize a liberty interest in refusing *life-sustaining* treatment because of the "dramatic consequences involved." When the chief justice hypothesized the existence of a competent person's liberty interest in refusing life-sustaining treatment, he did so *only* to identify the issue as *not* presented by this case.

Why would the chief justice hypothesize the existence of a liberty interest when its existence mattered not at all to the outcome of the case? Perhaps to satisfy the wishes of the fifth, and necessary, vote of Justice Sandra Day O'Connor. Justice O'Connor's concurring opinion makes clear that, though she provided a fifth vote for the outcome in this case, she was also a fifth vote willing to recognize a competent person's right to refuse life-sustaining treatment:

> I agree that a [constitutionally] protected liberty interest in refusing unwanted medical treatment may be inferred from our

prior decisions ... and that the refusal of artificially delivered food and water is encompassed within that liberty interest. I write separately to clarify why I believe this to be so. [p. 287]

What Chief Justice Rehnquist treated as hypothetical, Justice O'Connor treated as actual, and she presented her argument for its establishment.\* In the end she even spoke about the need to safeguard similar liberty interests for incompetents, giving shockingly little attention to the duty of the state to protect the life of incompetent people against those who would exercise on their behalf their putative right to die.\*\*

Only Justice Antonin Scalia, writing a concurring opinion, was willing to say (correctly, in my view) that the Constitution has absolutely nothing to say about this matter:

> What I have said above is not meant to suggest that I would think it desirable, if we were sure that Nancy Cruzan wanted to die, to keep her alive by the means at issue here. I only assert that the Constitution has nothing to say about the subject. To raise up a constitutional right here we would have to create out of nothing (for it exists neither in text nor tradition) some constitutional principle whereby, although the State may insist that

---

\*By the time the Court returned to this issue, even Chief Justice Rehnquist conceded that *Cruzan* stood for the right of a competent person to refuse treatment, even when that meant bringing about his own death (*Glucksberg*, p. 723). But it is important to note that the chief justice insisted that the right announced in *Cruzan* did *not* derive from some vague right to autonomy that the Constitution respects. Rather, the right to refuse medical treatment was firmly rooted in the common-law right to be free from battery, of which unwanted medical treatment was one instance.

\*\*Justice William Brennan, in his dissenting opinion, denies that the state has even a legitimate interest in—much less a duty toward—someone's life that could ever outweigh the person's choice to avoid medical treatment. And in the presence of a patient who can no longer choose for herself, the state has an interest *only* in trying to determine as accurately as possible "how she would exercise her rights under these circumstances.... [U]ntil Nancy's wishes have been determined, the only [!] state interest that may be asserted is an interest in safeguarding the accuracy of that determination" (*Cruzan*, 497 U.S. 261, pp. 315–16; emphasis in original). (This is, by the way, a seemingly impossible task, given the view of the self that is implicit in Justice Brennan's reasoning.) Not the security of life but the self-assertion of the self-determining will is, for Justice Brennan, the primary interest of the state. We see here how Nietzschean thinking threatens to replace classical American liberalism, even in constitutional interpretation.

an individual come in out of the cold and eat food, it may not insist that he take medicine; and although it may pump his stomach empty of poison he has ingested, it may not fill his stomach with food he has failed to ingest. [p. 300]

Yet paradoxically, Justice Scalia's powerful argument, which identified the refusal of food and water as suicide, could give ammunition to the other side, were it to be conjoined with the view of Justice O'Connor (and the four justices in the *Cruzan* minority) that a right to refuse *lifesaving* treatment is already constitutionally protected. Should Justice O'Connor's view prevail, Justice Scalia's argument could supply the reason for regarding the newly protected right implied in *Cruzan* as indeed a right to die. The elements were all in place for inventing a constitutional right to suicide and, in the case of incompetents, for assistance with suicide, that is, a full-fledged "right to die."

This, in fact, was precisely the tack taken in the two cases won by "right to die" plaintiffs in the United States Courts of Appeals for the Ninth and Second Circuits, both decided in 1996. Reading *Cruzan* as having tacitly provided for a qualified right to die, at least for a competent adult who is terminally ill, a group of physicians who treat terminally ill patients, joined by some of those patients, attacked statutory bans on assisted suicide in the states of Washington and New York. The doctors avowed that they would assist those gravely ill patients in ending their lives were it not for these bans. Arguing that these laws violated the Due Process and the Equal Protection Clauses of the Fourteenth Amendment, plaintiffs sought to convert the qualified "right to hasten one's death" through refusing life-sustaining treatment in *Cruzan* into an unqualified right to choose death directly through taking lethal drugs.* Next, because some patients are incapable of exercising their "right to die" on their own, plaintiffs argued for a constitutionally protected right to *assistance* in suicide.

Chief Justice Rehnquist, again writing for a majority of the Court, never let them take the first step. The proponents of assisted suicide had argued (from *Cruzan*) that a competent person has the

---

*The discussion here will focus on *Glucksberg*, the case that was argued on Due Process grounds, for it is here that a liberty interest in a right to die could be established. The *Quill* case raised Equal Protection arguments that do not really address the existence of such a right.

right to "hasten death," and that there is no difference between has-tening death by refusing medical treatment and hastening death by consuming lethal medication. Rehnquist rejected this analysis, con-cluding that there was, in fact, a big legal difference between the two. In doing so, he relied on the same narrow course he had set out in *Cruzan,* which rested not at all on lofty and unwieldy notions of privacy or a personal liberty to "hasten death," but on a narrow legal principle and a historical legal fact:

> the common law rule that forced medication was a battery, and the long legal tradition protecting the decision to refuse unwanted medical treatment.... The decision to commit sui-cide with the assistance of another may be just as personal and just as profound as the decision to refuse unwanted medical treatment, but it has never enjoyed similar legal protection. Indeed, the two acts are widely and reasonably regarded as quite distinct. [p. 725]

There was, Rehnquist insisted, no similar common-law tradition that might support a right to assisted suicide. Indeed, "[t]he history of the law's treatment of assisted suicide in this country has been and continues to be one of rejection of nearly all efforts to permit it" (p. 728). The lower court's decision establishing an unqualified right to become dead was here soundly rejected.

There is no doubt that the Supreme Court's decisions in *Glucks-berg* and *Quill* were a blow to the movement to establish a consti-tutional "right to die." Yet despite the unanimous verdicts, the door has been left open. Once again, only five justices signed the major-ity opinion, the rest concurring on different grounds. And once again, Justice O'Connor muddied the waters. As in *Cruzan,* she signed the chief justice's opinion to make it a majority opinion, but this time she also wrote separately in ways that cast doubt on the degree to which she actually holds with the majority she helped to form. Incon-sistencies between her short concurrence and the majority opinion abound.* She agrees with the majority, she says, because she agrees "that there is no *generalized right* to 'commit suicide'" (p. 736;

---

*\**Glucksberg,* 521 U.S. 736 (O'Connor, J. concurring). Justice Stephen Breyer joined Justice O'Connor's opinion, *except insofar as she joined the Court's opinion,* a fact suggesting a tension between the two.

emphasis added), but this was *not* the main question in the case; indeed, it was not even a position argued by anyone in the case. She sees no reason to reach what she calls "the narrower question," the question that was in fact at issue in the case: "whether a mentally competent person who is experiencing great suffering has a constitutionally cognizable interest in controlling the circumstances of his or her *imminent death*" (p. 736; emphasis added). Apparently reserving the right to decide *this* question at a later time, Justice O'Connor does not explain how this position can be reconciled with the majority opinion she also signed. For the majority had clearly held that there is no basis in the legal tradition for finding *any* constitutionally defensible exception to bans on assisted suicide for those who are near to death.

How to explain these various imprecisions and inconsistencies? Yale Kamisar offers a likely suggestion:

> What is the most plausible explanation for Justice O'Connor's odd statement that she is joining the chief justice's opinions in *Glucksberg* and *Quill* because she "agree[s] that there is no generalized right to 'commit suicide'?" Although it is a conclusion that I am not eager to reach, I think the reason for Justice O'Connor's statement is a reluctance to rule out the possibility of a right to physician-assisted suicide in every set of circumstances and a desire to "proceed with caution" in this area.[14]

This suggestion is supported by yet more disquieting language in her discussion of the role of state legislatures in grappling with these complex end-of-life decisions.

Justice O'Connor, like the majority, recognized that "States are presently undertaking extensive and serious evaluation of physician assisted suicide and other related issues" (p. 737). To Rehnquist, this is as it should be "in a democratic society" (p. 735) End of matter. To Justice O'Connor, though, this means that the "challenging task of crafting appropriate procedures for safeguarding ... *liberty interests* is entrusted to the laboratory of the states ... *in the first instance*" (p. 737; emphasis added). Wait a minute. *What* liberty interest? A reader of Rehnquist's opinion would have thought there was no liberty interest in "hastening death" at stake here. "In the first instance"?

That is more than a little foreboding. Justice O'Connor stands ready to ensure that those state laboratories ultimately get it *right*.

We should therefore not be overly confident that we have heard the end of claims to a constitutional "right to die." This cryptic concurrence by a member of a five-vote majority can only undermine the precedential standing of Rehnquist's otherwise clear opinion. As with all judicial opinions, the meaning of this opinion is left to a later Court (potentially made up of different personnel) to decide. Justice O'Connor's concurrence, imprecise in what little it says, may well serve only one purpose: provide a future "swing" justice with the wiggle room to get out from under Rehnquist's opinion so that he or she may do whatever he or she thinks best and "establish" by judicial usurpation a constitutional "right to die."

## The Tragic Meaning of "Right to Die"

The claim of a "right to die," asserted especially against physicians bent on prolonging life, clearly exposes certain deep difficulties in the foundations of modern society. Modern liberal, technological society rests especially upon two philosophical pillars raised first in the seventeenth century, at the beginning of the modern era: the pre-eminence of the human individual, embodied in the doctrine of natural rights as espoused first by Hobbes and Locke; and the idea of mastery of nature, attained through a radically new science of nature as proposed by Francis Bacon and René Descartes.

Both ideas were responses to the perceived partial inhospitality of nature to human need. Both encouraged man's opposition to nature: the first through the flight from the state of nature into civil society for the purpose of safeguarding the precarious rights to life and liberty; the second through the subduing of nature for the purpose of making life longer, healthier and more commodious. One might even say it is especially an opposition to death that grounds these twin responses. Politically, the fear of violent death at the hands of warring men requires law and legitimate authority to secure natural rights, especially life. Technologically, the fear of death as such at the hands of unfriendly nature inspires a bolder approach, namely, a scientific medicine to wage war against disease and even against death itself, ultimately with a promise of bodily immortality.

Drunk on its political and scientific successes, modern thought and practice have abandoned the modest and moderate beginnings of political modernity. In civil society the natural rights of self-preservation, secured through active but moderate self-assertion, have given way to the non-natural rights of self-creation and self-expression; the new rights have no connection to nature or to reason, but appear as the rights of the untrammeled will. The "self" that here asserts itself is not a natural self, with the predictable interests given to it by a universal human nature with its bodily needs, but a uniquely individuated and self-made self. Its authentic selfhood is demonstrated by its ability to say no to the needs of the body, the rules of society and the dictates of reason. For such a self, self-negation through suicide and the right to die can be the ultimate form of self-assertion.

In medical science, the unlimited battle against death has found nature unwilling to roll over and play dead. The successes of medicine so far are partial at best and the victory incomplete, to say the least. The welcome triumphs against disease have been purchased at the price of the medicalized dehumanization of the end of life: to put it starkly, once we lick cancer and stroke, we can all live long enough to get Alzheimer's disease. And if the insurance holds out, we can die in the intensive care unit, suitably intubated. Fear of the very medical power we engaged to do battle against death now leads us to demand that it give us poison.

Finally, both the triumph of individualism and our reliance on technology (not only in medicine) and on government to satisfy our new wants-demanded-as-rights have weakened our more natural human associations—especially the family, on which we all need to rely when our pretense to autonomy and mastery is eventually exposed by unavoidable decline. Old age and death have been taken out of the bosom of family life and turned over to state-supported nursing homes and hospitals. Not the clergyman but the doctor (in truth, the nurse) presides over the end of life, in sterile surroundings that make no concessions to our finitude. Both the autonomous will and the will's partner in pride, the death-denying doctor, ignore the unavoidable limits on will and technique that nature insists on.

Failure to recognize these limits now threatens the entire venture; for rebellion against the project through a "right to die" will only radicalize its difficulties. Vulnerable life will no longer be protected by the state, medicine will become a death-dealing profession, and isolated individuals will be technically dispatched to avoid the troubles of finding human ways to keep company with them in their time of ultimate need.

That the right to die should today be asserted to win release from a hyperpowerful medical futility is thus more than tragic irony; it is also very dangerous. Three dangers especially stand out.

First, the right to die, especially as it comes to embrace a right to "aid-in-dying," or assisted suicide, or euthanasia, will translate into an obligation on the part of others to kill or help kill. Even if we refuse to impose such a duty but merely allow those others who are freely willing, our society would be drastically altered. For unless the state accepts the job of euthanizer—which God forbid that it should—it would thus surrender its monopoly on the legal use of lethal force, a monopoly it holds and needs if it is to protect innocent life, its first responsibility.

Second, there can be no way to confine the practice to those who knowingly and freely request death. The vast majority of persons who are candidates for assisted death are, and will increasingly be, incapable of choosing and effecting such a course of action for themselves. No one with an expensive or troublesome infirmity will be safe from the pressure to have his right to die exercised.

Third, the medical profession's devotion to heal and refusal to kill—its ethical center—will be permanently destroyed, and with it, patient trust and physicianly self-restraint. Here is yet another case where acceding to a putative personal right would wreak havoc on the common good.

Nothing I have said should be taken to mean that I believe life should be extended under all circumstances and at all costs. Far from it. I continue, with fear and trembling, to defend the practice of allowing to die while opposing the practice of deliberately killing— despite the blurring of this morally bright line implicit in the case of artificial nutrition, and despite the slide toward the retailing of death that continues on the sled of a right to refuse treatment. I welcome efforts to give patients as much choice as possible in how they are to live out the end of their lives. I continue to applaud those courageous patients and family members and those conscientious physicians who try prudently to discern, in each case, just what form of treatment or nontreatment is truly good for the patient, even if it embraces an increased likelihood of death. But I continue to insist that we cannot serve the patient's good by deliberately eliminating the patient. And if we have no right to do this to another, we have no right to have others do this to ourselves. There is, when all is said and done, no defensible right to die.

## A Coda: About Rights

The rhetoric of rights still performs today the noble, time-honored function of protecting individual life and liberty, a function now perhaps even more necessary than the originators of such rhetoric could have imagined, given the tyrannical possibilities of the modern bureaucratic and technologically competent state. But with the claim of a "right to die," as with so many of the novel rights being asserted in recent years, we face an extension of this rhetoric into areas where it no longer relates to that protective function, and beyond the limited area of life in which rights claims are clearly appropriate and indeed crucial. As a result, we face a number of serious and potentially dangerous distortions in our thought and in our practice. We distort our understanding of rights and weaken their respectability in their proper sphere by allowing them to be invented—without ground in nature or in reason—in response to moral questions that lie outside the limited domain of rights. We distort our understanding of moral deliberation and the moral life by reducing all complicated questions of right and good to questions of individual rights. We subvert the primacy and necessity of prudence by pretending that the assertion of rights will produce the best—and most moral—results. In trying to batter our way through the human condition with the bludgeon of personal rights, we allow ourselves to be deceived about the most fundamental matters: about death and dying, about our unavoidable finitude, and about the sustaining interdependencies of our lives.

Let us, by all means, continue to deliberate about whether and when and why it might make sense for someone to give up on his life, or even actively to choose death. But let us call a halt to all this dangerous thoughtlessness about rights. Let us, specifically, refuse to talk any longer about a "right to die."

# CHAPTER EIGHT

# Death with Dignity and the Sanctity of Life

Dispatching the claims of a "right to die" helps us to avoid great mischief. It also reminds us that we cannot bring the mystery of death under the control of human will and self-assertion. Yet it leaves us with those who are dying and the dilemmas involved in their proper care. It also leaves us with the need to ponder how the end of life should relate to the rest of it.

"Call no man happy until he's dead." So did the ancient Athenian sage Solon remind the self-satisfied Croesus of the perils of fortune and the need to see the end of a life before pronouncing on its happiness. Even the richest man on earth has little control over his fate. The unpredictability of human life is an old story; many a once-flourishing life has ended in years of debility, dependence and disgrace. But today, it seems, the problems of the ends of lives are more acute, a consequence, ironically, of successful—or partly successful—human efforts to do battle with fortune and, in particular, to roll back medically the causes of death. While many look forward to further triumphs in the war against mortality, others here and now want to exercise greater control over the end of life, by electing death to avoid the burdens of lingering on. The failures resulting from the fight against fate are to be resolved by taking fate still further into our own hands.

This is no joking matter. Nor are the questions it raises academic. They emerge, insistently and urgently, from poignant human situations, occurring daily in hospitals and nursing homes, as patients and families and physicians are compelled to decide matters of life and death, often in the face only of unattractive, even horrible, alternatives. Shall I allow the doctors to put a feeding tube into my eighty-five-year-old mother, who is unable to swallow as a result of a stroke?

Now that it is inserted and she is not recovering, may I have it removed? When would it be right to remove a respirator, forego renal dialysis, bypass lifesaving surgery, or omit giving antibiotics for pneumonia? When in the course of my own progressive dementia will it be right for my children to put me into a home or for me to ask my doctor or my wife or my daughter for a lethal injection? When, if ever, should I as a physician or husband or son accede to— or be forgiven for acceding to—such a request?

These dilemmas can be multiplied indefinitely, and their human significance is hard to capture in words. For one thing, posing them as well-defined problems to be solved subtracts from the full human picture, and ignores such matters as the relations between the generations, the meaning of old age, attitudes toward mortality, religious faith, economic resources, and the like. Also, speech doesn't begin to convey the anguish and heartache felt by those who concretely confront such terrible decisions, nor can it do much to aid and comfort them. Moreover, any generalized discussion necessarily abstracts from the special and concrete features of each human situation. No amount of philosophizing is going to substitute for discernment, compassion, courage, sobriety, tact, thoughtfulness or prudence, all needed on the spot.

Yet the attitudes, sentiments and judgments of human agents on the spot are influenced, often unwittingly, by speech and opinion, and by the terms in which we formulate our concerns. Some speech may illuminate, other speech may distort; some terms may be more or less appropriate to the matter at hand. About death and dying, once subjects treated with decorous or superstitious silence, there is today an abundance of talk—not to say indecorous chatter. Moreover, this talk frequently proceeds under the aegis of certain increasingly accepted terminologies, which are, in my view, both questionable in themselves and dangerous in their influence. As a result, we are producing a recipe for disaster: Urgent difficulties, great human anguish, high emotions stirred up with inadequate thinking. We have no choice but to reflect on our speech and our terminology.

In the last chapter I showed how the notion of "rights" has confused our current discussions about death and dying. The idea of "duty" has done comparable mischief. From the acknowledged human duty not to shed innocent blood follows the public duty to protect life against those who would threaten it. This gets extended to a duty to preserve life in the face of disease or other nonhuman dangers to life. This gets extended to a duty to prolong life whenever possible, regardless of the condition of that life or the wishes of its bearer. This gets extended to an unconditional duty never to let death happen, if it lies in one's power to do so. This position, sometimes alleged—I think mistakenly—to be entailed by belief in the "sanctity of life," could even make obligatory a search for the conquest of death altogether, through research on aging (see Chapter Nine). Do we have such duties? On what do they rest? And can such a duty to prevent death—or a right to life—be squared with a right to be made dead? Is not this intransigent language of rights and duties unsuitable for finding the best course of action, in these terribly ambiguous and weighty matters? We must try to become more thoughtful about the terms we use and the questions we pose.

Toward this end I explore in this chapter the relation between two powerful notions, both prominent in the discussions regarding the end of life: death with dignity, and the sanctity of life. Both convey elevated, indeed lofty, ideas: what, after all, could be higher than human dignity, unless it were something sacred? As a result, each phrase often functions as a slogan or a rallying cry, though seldom with any regard for its meaning or ground. In the current debates about euthanasia, we are often told that these notions pull in opposite directions. Upholding death with dignity might mean taking actions that would seem to deny the sanctity of life. Conversely, unswervingly upholding the sanctity of life might mean denying to some a dignified death. This implied opposition is, for many of us, very disquieting. The dilemmas themselves are bad enough. Much worse is it to contemplate that human dignity and sanctity might be opposed, and that we may be forced to choose between them.*

---

*Some people, in contrast, are delighted with this polarized framing of the question, for they see it as the conflict between a vigorous humanism and an anachronistic otherworldliness foisted upon the West by the Judeo-Christian tradition. For those who deny the sacred, it is desirable to represent the arguments against suicide or mercy killing (or abortion) as purely religious in character—there being, in their view, nothing higher than human dignity. The chief proponent of a "Humane and Dignified Death Initiative" in California in the late 1980s is reported to have said that he was seeking to "overturn the sanctity of life principle" in American law.

The confrontation between upholders of death with dignity and upholders of the sanctity of life is nothing new. Three decades ago, the contest was over termination of treatment and letting die. Today the issue is the "right to die" and assisted suicide. Tomorrow it will be the "duty to die" and mercy killing (so-called active euthanasia). On the extremes of both battles stand the same opponents, many of whom—I think mistakenly—think the issues are the same. Many who now oppose mercy killing or voluntary euthanasia then opposed termination of treatment, thinking it equivalent to killing. Those who today back mercy killing in fact agree: if it is permissible to choose death by letting die, they argue, why not also by active steps to hasten, humanely, the desired death? Failing to distinguish between letting die and making dead (by failing to distinguish between intentions and motives, causes and results, goals and outcomes), both sides polarize the debate, opposing not only one another but also those in the uncomfortable middle. For them, it is *either* sanctity of life *or* death with dignity; one must choose.

I do not accept this polarization. In the rest of this chapter I mean to suggest the following: First, human dignity and the sanctity of life not only are compatible, but if rightly understood, they go hand in hand. Second, death with dignity, rightly understood, has largely to do with exercising the humanity that life makes possible, often to the very end, and very little to do with medical procedures or the causes of death. Third, the sanctity-and-dignity of life is entirely compatible with letting die but not with deliberately killing. Finally, the practice of euthanasia does not conduce to human dignity and our rush to embrace it will only accelerate the various tendencies in our society that undermine not only dignified conduct but even decent human relations.

## The Sanctity of Life (and Human Dignity)

What exactly is meant by the sanctity of life? This turns out to be difficult to say. In the strictest sense, sanctity of life would mean that life is *in itself* something holy or sacred, transcendent, set apart—like God himself. Or, again, to begin with our responses to the sacred, it would mean that life is something before which we stand (or should stand) with reverence, awe and grave respect—because it is beyond us and unfathomable. In more modest but also more practical terms, to regard life as sacred means that it should not be violated, opposed or destroyed, and, positively, that it should be protected, defended and preserved. Despite their differences, these various formulations agree in this: that "sacredness," whatever it is, inheres in life itself, and that life, *by its very being,* calls forth an appropriate human response, whether of veneration or restraint. To say that sacredness is something that can be conferred or ascribed—or removed—by solely human agreement or decision is to miss the point entirely.

Yet there is further difficulty. Which or what life is sacred: only human life or animal (and plant) life also? If the latter, is animal life sacred equally with human life, or can there be degrees of "sanctity"? And within human life, is it the individuated being, the conscious or rational being, or the whole organism simply as human whose life is sacred? Is the lineage holy, or the race or the nation or the species? Or is it not life as such but life lived in a certain way, for example, the life according to the Torah, that has sanctity?

A deeper question: What is the ground or basis of life's sanctity? Does it depend decisively on a divine act, either that life was made by God or that He later sanctified it (as He did the Sabbath)? Or, quite apart from its origins, is there perhaps something godlike about life or human life (for example, spirit), which calls forth awe and respect, and before which we stand somewhat as we do before the divine? More experientially, leaving all revelation to one side, is there not something "protoreligious" in the joyous experience of birth, in the horror of extinction, and in many of the astonishing appearances and doings of all living things, before which the proper response is wondering-awe? What is it that makes what kind of life sacred? Just raising these questions shows how difficult it would be, philosophically, to understand the sanctity of life.

To the best of my knowledge, the phrase "sanctity of life" does not occur either in the Hebrew Bible or in the New Testament. Life as such is not said to be holy (*qadosh*), as is, for example, the Sabbath. The Jewish people are said to be a holy people, and they are enjoined to be holy as God is holy. True, traditional Judaism places great emphasis on preserving human life—even the holy Sabbath may be violated to save a life, implying to some that a human life is more to be revered than the Sabbath—yet the duty to preserve one's life is not unconditional: to cite only one example, a Jew should accept martyrdom rather than commit idolatry, adultery or murder.

As murder would be the most direct assault on human life and the most explicit denial of its sanctity, perhaps we gain some access to the meaning of the sanctity of life by thinking about why murder is proscribed. If we could uncover the ground of restraint against murder, perhaps we could learn something about the nature of the sanctity of life, and perhaps also about its relation to human dignity. As a result, we might be in a better position to consider the propriety of letting die, of euthanasia, and of other activities sometimes embraced by the adherents of "death with dignity."

Why is killing another human being wrong? Can the prospective victim's request to be killed nullify the wrongness of such killing, or, what's more, make such killing right? Alternatively, are there specifiable states or conditions of a human being's life that would justify—or excuse—someone else's directly and intentionally putting him to death, even *without* request? The first question asks about murder, the second and third ask whether assisting suicide and mercy killing can and should be morally distinguished from murder. The answers regarding assisting suicide and euthanasia will depend on the answer regarding murder, that is, on the *reasons* why it is wrong.*

Why is murder wrong? The laws against murder are, of course, socially useful. Though murders still occur, despite the proscriptive

---

*Not all taking of human life is murder. Self-defense, war and capital punishment have been moral grounds used to justify homicide, and it is a rare moralist who would argue that it is never right to kill another human being. Without arguing about these exceptions, we confine our attention to murder, which by definition is unjust or wrongful killing. Everyone knows it to be wrong, immediately and without argument. Rarely do we ask ourselves why.

This is, of course, as it should be. The most important insights on which decent society rests—for example, the taboos against incest, cannibalism, murder and adultery—are too important to be imperiled by reason's poor power to give them convincing defense. Such taboos might themselves be the incarnation of reason, even as they resist attempts to give them logical demonstration; like the axioms of geometry, they might be at once incapable of proof and yet not in need of proof, that is, self-evident to anyone not morally blind. What follows, then, is more a search for insight than an attempt at proof.

law and the threat of punishment, civil society is possible only because people generally accept and abide by the reasonableness of this rule. In exchange for society's protection of one's own life against those who might otherwise take it away, each member of society sacrifices, in principle, his (natural) right to the lives of all others. Civil society requires peace, and civil peace depends absolutely on the widespread adherence to the maxim, "Thou shalt not murder." This usefulness of the taboo against murder is sometimes offered as the basis of its goodness: killing is bad because it makes life unsafe and society impossible.

But this alone cannot account for the taboo against murder. In fact, the goodness of civil society is itself predicated upon the goodness of human life, which society is instituted to defend and foster. Civil society exists to defend the goods implicit in the taboo against murder, at least as much as the taboo against murder is useful in preserving civil society.

However valuable any life may be to the society, each life is primarily and preeminently valued by the person whose life it is. Individuals strive to stay alive, both consciously and unconsciously. The living body, quite on its own, bends every effort to maintain its living existence. Built-in impulses toward self-preservation and individual well-being penetrate our consciousness; hunger and fear of death, for example, are manifestations of a deep-seated and powerful will-to-live. These thoughts might suggest that murder is wrong because it opposes this will-to-live, because it deprives another of life against his will, because it kills someone who does not *want* to die. This sort of reason would explain why suicide—self-willed self-killing—might be right, while murder—killing an innocent person against his will—would always be wrong.

Let us consider this view more closely. Certainly, there are some invasions or "violations" of another's body that are made innocent by consent. Blows struck in a boxing match or on the football field do not constitute assault; conversely, an unwelcome kiss from a stranger, because it is an unconsented touching, constitutes a battery, actionable at law. In these cases, the willingness or unwillingness of the "victim" alone determines the rightness or wrongness of the bodily impact. Similar arguments are today used to explain the wrongness of rape: it is "against our wills," a violation not (as we once thought) of womanliness or chastity or nature but of freedom, autonomy, personal self-determination. If consent excuses—or even justifies—these "attacks" on the body of another, might not consent excuse—or justify—the ultimate, that is, lethal, attack and turn murder into merely (unwrongful) homicide? A person can be murdered only if he personally does not want to be dead.

There is something obviously troublesome in this way of thinking about crimes against persons. Indeed, the most abominable practices, proscribed in virtually all societies, are *not* excused by consent. Incest, even between consenting adults, is still incest; cannibalism would not become merely *delicatessen* if the victim freely gave permission; ownership of human beings, voluntarily accepted, would still be slavery. The violation of the other is independent of the state of the will (in fact, of both victim and perpetrator).

The questions can be put this way: Is the life of another human being to be respected only because that person (or society) *deems* or *wills* it respectable, or is it to be respected because it *is in itself* respectable? If the former, then human worth depends solely on agreement or human will; since will confers dignity, will can take it away, and permission to violate nullifies the violation. If the latter, then one can never be released from the obligation to respect human life by a request to do so, say, from someone who no longer values his own life.

This latter view squares best with our intuitions. We are not entitled to dismember the corpse of a suicide nor may we kill innocently those consumed by self-hatred. According to our law, killing the willing, the unwilling and the nonwilling (for example, infants or the comatose) are all equally murder. Beneath the human will, indeed, the *ground* of human will, is something that commands respect and restraint, willy-nilly. We are to abstain from killing because of something respectable about human beings as such. But what is it?

In Western societies, moral notions trace back to biblical religion. The bedrock of Jewish and Christian morality is the Ten Commandments. "Thou shalt not murder"—the sixth commandment—heads up the so-called second table, which enunciates (negatively) duties toward one's fellow man. From this fact, some people have argued that murder is wrong solely because God said so. After all, that He had to legislate against it might imply that human beings on their own did not know that it was bad or wrong. Even were they to intuit *that* murder is wrong, they might never be able to answer, if challenged, *why* it is wrong, and this human inability to supply the reason would threaten the power of the taboo. Thus, so the argument goes, God's will supplies the missing reason for the human rule.

This argument is not satisfactory. True, divine authority elevates the standing and force of the commandments; yet it does not follow that they "make sense" only because God willed them. Pagans yesterday believed and atheists today still believe that murder is wrong. And while the latter might be suspected of being under the influence of a morality whose source they reject, other cultures and other nonreligious thinkers line up squarely against murder. Aristotle, who did not know of the biblical God, spoke for rationality itself when he said that the very name "murder"—like adultery and theft—implies badness. In fact, the entire second table of the Decalogue is said to propound not so much divine law but natural law, suitable for man as man, not only for Jew or Christian.

The Bible itself could be said to provide evidence in support of this interpretation, at least about murder. It reports that after the first murder, committed by Cain upon his brother Abel before there was any given or known law against it, Abel's blood cried out from the earth in protest against his brother's deed. (The crime, it seems, was a crime against blood and life, not against will, human or divine.) And Cain's denial of knowledge ("Am I my brother's keeper?") seems a clear indication of guilt: if there were nothing wrong with murder, why hide one's responsibility? A "protoreligious" dread accompanies the encounter with death, especially violent death.

But the best evidence comes shortly afterward, in the story of the covenant with Noah: the first law against murder is explicitly promulgated for all mankind united, well before there are Jews or Christians or Muslims. This passage is worth looking at in some detail because, unlike the enunciation of the sixth commandment, it offers a specific reason why murder is wrong.*

---

*Nonreligious readers may rightly express suspicion at my appeal to a biblical text for what I will claim is a universal or philosophical explanation of the taboo against murder. This suspicion will be further increased by the content of the text cited. Nevertheless, properly interpreted, I believe the teaching of the passage stands free of its especially biblical roots, and offers a profound insight into the ground of our respect for human life.

The prohibition of murder—or, to be more precise, the institution of retribution for shedding human blood—is part of the new order following the Flood. Before the Flood, human beings lived in the absence of law or civil society. The result appears to be something like what Hobbes called the state of nature, characterized as a condition of war of each against all. Might alone makes right, and no one is safe. The Flood washes out human life in its natural state; immediately afterward, some form of law and justice is instituted, and nascent civil society is founded.

At the forefront of the new order is a newly articulated respect for human life,* expressed in the announcement of the punishment for homicide: "Whoso sheddeth man's blood, by man shall his blood be shed; for in the image of God made He man." (Genesis 9:6) Like law in general, this cardinal law combines speech and force. The threat of capital punishment stands as a deterrent to murder and hence provides a motive for obedience. But the measure of the punishment is instructive. By stipulating a life for a life—no *more* than a life for a life, and that only of the murderer, not also of his wife and children, for example—the threatened punishment implicitly teaches the *equal* worth of each human life. Such equality can be grounded only in the equal *humanity* of each human being. Against our own native self-preference, and against our tendency to overvalue what is our own, blood-for-blood conveys the message of universality and equality.

But murder is to be avoided not only to avoid the punishment. That may be a motive, which speaks to our fears; but there is also a reason, which speaks to our minds and our loftier sentiments. The fundamental reason that makes murder wrong—and that even

---

*This respect for human life, and the self-conscious establishment of society on this premise, separates human beings from the rest of the animals. This separation is made emphatic by the institution of meat eating (Genesis 9:1–4), permitted to men here for the first time. (One can, I believe, show that the permission to eat meat is a concession to human blood lust and voracity, not something cheerfully and happily endorsed.) Yet, curiously, even animal life must be treated with respect: the blood, which is identified as the life, cannot be consumed. Human life, as we shall see more clearly, is thus both continuous and discontinuous with animal life.

justifies punishing it homicidally!—is man's divine-like status.* Not
the other fellow's unwillingness to be killed, not even (or only) our
desire to avoid sharing his fate, but *his*—any man's—*very being*
requires that we respect his life. Human life is to be respected more
than animal life, because man is more than an animal; man is said
to be godlike. Please note that the *truth* of the Bible's assertion does
*not* rest on biblical authority: man's more-than-animal status is in
fact performatively proved whenever human beings quit the state
of nature and set up life under such a law. The law establishing that
men are to be law-abiding both insists on, and thereby demonstrates
the truth of, the superiority of man.

How is man godlike? Genesis 1—where it is first said that man
is created in God's image—introduces us to the divine *activities* and
*powers:* (1) God speaks, commands, names and blesses; (2) God
makes and makes freely; (3) God looks at and beholds the world;
(4) God is concerned with the goodness or perfection of things; (5)
God addresses solicitously other living creatures. In short: God exer-
cises speech and reason, freedom in doing and making, and the powers of contemplation, judgment and care.

Doubters may wonder whether this is truly the case about
God—after all, it is only on biblical authority that we regard God
as possessing these powers and activities. But it is certain that we
human beings have them, and that they lift us above the plane of a
merely animal existence. Human beings, alone among the earthly
creatures, speak, plan, create, contemplate and judge. Human beings,
alone among the creatures, can articulate a future goal and bring it
into being by their own purposive conduct. Human beings, alone
among the creatures, can think about the whole, marvel at its articulated order, and feel awe in beholding its grandeur and in pondering the mystery of its source.

A complementary, preeminently moral, gloss on the "image of
God" is provided—quite explicitly—in Genesis 3, at the end of the
so-called second creation story: "Now the man is become *like one*

---

*The second part of verse 6 seems to make two points: man is in the image of God
(that is, godlike), and man was made thus by God. The decisive point is the first.
Man's creatureliness cannot be the reason for avoiding bloodshed; the animals too
were made by God, yet permission to kill them for food has just been given. The full
weight rests on man's *being* "in the image of God."

*of us* knowing good and bad...." (3:22; emphasis added.)* Human beings, unlike the other animals, distinguish good and bad, have opinions and care about their difference, and constitute their whole life in the light of this distinction. Animals may suffer good and bad, but they have no notion of either. Indeed, the very pronouncement, "Murder is bad," constitutes proof of *this* godlike quality of human beings.

In sum, man has special standing because he shares in reason, freedom, judgment and moral concern, and as a result, he lives a life freighted with moral self-consciousness. Speech and freedom are used, among other things, to promulgate moral rules and to pass moral judgments, first among which is that murder is to be punished in kind because it violates the dignity of such a moral being. We note a crucial implication: simply put, the *sanctity* of human life rests absolutely on the *dignity*—the godlikeness—of human beings.

Yet man is, at most, only godly; he is not God or a god. To be an image is also to be *different* from that of which one is an image. Man is, at most, a *mere* likeness of God. With us, the seemingly godly powers and concerns described above occur conjoined with our animality. We are also flesh and blood—no less than the other animals. God's image is tied to blood, which is the life.

The point is crucial, and stands apart from the text that teaches it: everything high about human life—thinking, judging, loving, willing, acting—depends absolutely on everything low—metabolism, digestion, respiration, circulation, excretion. In the case of human beings, "divinity" needs blood—or "mere" life—to sustain itself. And because of what it holds up, human blood—that is, human life—deserves special respect, beyond what is owed to life as such; the low ceases to be the low. (Modern physiological evidence could be adduced in support of this thesis: in human beings, posture, gestalt, respiration, sexuality, and fetal and infant development, among other things, all show the marks of the co-presence of rationality.) The biblical text elegantly mirrors this truth about its subject, subtly merging both high and low: though the reason

---

*In the first creation story, Genesis 1–2:3, man is created straightaway in God's likeness; in this second account, man is, to begin with, made of dust, and he *acquires* godlike qualities only at the end, and then only in transgressing.

given for punishing murder concerns man's godliness, the injunction itself concerns man's blood. Respect the godlike; don't shed its blood! Respect for anything human requires respecting *everything* human, requires respecting *human being* as such.

We have found, I believe, what we were searching for: a reason immanent in the nature of things for finding fault with taking human life, apart from the needs of society or the will of the victim. The wanton spilling of human blood is a violation and a desecration, not only of our laws and wills but of our being itself.

We have also found the ground for repudiating the opposition between the sanctity of life and human dignity. Each rests on the other. Or, rather, they are mutually implicated, as inseparable as the concave and the convex. Those who seek to pull them apart are, I submit, also engaged in wanton, albeit intellectual, violence.

Unfortunately, the matter cannot simply rest here. Though the principle seems well established, there is a difficulty, raised in fact by the text itself. How can one assert the inviolability of human life and, in the same breath, insist that human beings deliberately *take* human life to punish those who shed human blood?* There are, it seems, sometimes good reasons for shedding human blood, notwithstanding that man is in God's image. We have admitted the dangerous principle: humanity, to uphold the dignity of the human, must sometimes shed human blood.

Bringing this new principle to the case of euthanasia, we face the following challenge to the prior, and more fundamental, principle: Shed no human blood. What are we to think when the continuing circulation of human blood no longer holds up anything very

---

*Does this mean that those who murder forfeit their claim to be humanly respected, because they implicitly have denied the humanity of their victim (and thus, in principle, of their own—and all other—human life)? In other words, do men need to act in accordance with the self-knowledge of human godliness in order to be treated accordingly? Or, conversely, do we rather respect the humanity of murderers when we punish them, even capitally, treating them not as crazed or bestial but as responsible moral agents who accept the fair consequences of their deeds? Or is the capitalness of the punishment not a theoretic matter, but a practical one, intended mainly to deter by fear those whose self-love or will-to-power will not listen to reason? These are vexed questions, too complicated to sort out quickly, and, in any case, beyond the point of the present discussion. Yet the relevant difficulty persists.

high, when it holds up little more—or even *no* more—than metabolism, digestion, respiration, circulation and excretion? What if human godliness appears to be humiliated by the degradation of Alzheimer's disease or paraplegia or rampant malignancy? And what if it is the well-considered aspiration of the "godlike" to put an end to the humiliation of that very godliness, to halt the mockery that various severe debilities make of a *human* life? Are there here to be found other exceptions to our rule against murder, in which the dignity of a human life can (only?) be respected by ending it?

The first thing to observe, of course, is that the cases of euthanasia (or suicide) and capital punishment are vastly different. One cannot by an act of euthanasia deter or correct or obtain justice from the "violator" of human dignity; senility and terminal illness are of natural origin and can be blamed on no human agent. To be precise, these evils may in their result undermine human dignity, but, lacking malevolent intention, cannot be said to insult it or deny it. They are reasons for sadness, not indignation, unless one believes, as the tyrant does, that the cosmos owes him good and not evil and exists to satisfy his every wish. Moreover, one does not come to the defense of diminished human dignity by finishing the job, by annihilating the victim. Human dignity would be no more vindicated by euthanizing patients with Alzheimer's disease than it would by executing as polluted the victims of rape.

Nevertheless, the question persists, and an affirmative answer remains the point of departure for the active euthanasia movement. Many who fly the banner of "death with dignity" insist that it centrally includes the option of active euthanasia, especially when requested. In order to respond more adequately to this challenge, we need first a more careful inquiry into "death with dignity."

## *Death with Dignity*

The phrase "death with dignity," whatever it means precisely, certainly implies that there are more and less dignified ways to die. The demand for death with dignity arises only because more and more people are encountering in others and fearing for themselves or their loved ones the deaths of the less dignified sort. This point is indisputable. The possibility of dying with dignity can be diminished or undermined by many things, for example, by coma or senility or madness, by unbearable pain or extensive paralysis, by isolation or rejection, by institutionalization or destitution, by sudden death, as well as by excessive or impersonal medical interventions directed toward the postponement of death. It is the impediments connected with modern medicine that increasingly arouse indignation, and the demand for death with dignity pleads for the removal of these "unnatural" obstacles.

More generally, the demand for autonomy and the cry for dignity are asserted against a medicalization and institutionalization of the end of life that robs the old and the incurable of most of their autonomy and dignity: intubated and electrified, with bizarre mechanical companions, confined and immobile, helpless and regimented, once proud and independent people find themselves cast in the roles of passive, obedient, highly disciplined children. Death with dignity means, in the first instance, the removal of these added indignities and dehumanizations of the end of life.

One can only sympathize with this concern. Yet even if successful, efforts to remove these obstacles would not yet produce a death with dignity. For one thing, not all obstacles to dignity are artificial and externally imposed. Infirmity and incompetence, dementia and immobility—all of them of natural origin—greatly limit human possibility, and for many of us they will be sooner or later unavoidable, the products of inevitable bodily or mental decay. Second, there is nothing of human dignity in the process of dying itself, only in the way we face it. At its best, death with complete dignity will always be compromised by extinction of dignified humanity; it is, I suspect, a death-denying culture's anger about dying and mortality that expresses itself in the partly oxymoronic and unreasonable demand for dignity in death. Third, insofar as we seek better health and longer life, insofar as we turn to doctors to help us get better, we necessarily and voluntarily compromise our dignity: being a patient rather than an agent is, humanly speaking, undignified. All people, especially the old, willingly, if unknowingly, accept a whole stable of indignities simply by seeking medical assistance. The really proud people refuse altogether to submit to doctors and hospitals. It is well to be reminded of these limits on our ability to roll back the indignities that assault the dying, so that we might acquire more realistic expectations about just how much dignity a "death-with-dignity" campaign can provide.

A death with positive dignity—which may turn out to be something rare, like a life with dignity—entails more than the absence of external indignities. Dignity in the face of death cannot be given or conferred from the outside; it requires a dignity of soul in the human being who faces it. This—despite the many claims to the contrary—neither the partisans of "death with dignity" nor the myriad servants of mankind, from the Department of Health and Human Services to departments of medicine or psychiatry, can supply, although they can, perhaps, offer some assistance. The following distinction seems roughly apt: we might say that the possibility of a humanly dignified facing of death can be destroyed or undermined from without (and, of course, from within), but the actualization of that possibility depends largely on the soul, the character, the bearing of the dying man himself—that is, on things within. To understand the meaning of and prospects for death with dignity, we need first to think more about dignity itself, what it is.

Dignity is, to begin with, an undemocratic idea. The central notion etymologically, both in English and in its Latin root (*dignitas*),* is that of worthiness, elevation, honor, nobility, height—in short, excellence or virtue. In all its meanings it is a term of distinction. Dignity is not something which, like a nose or a navel, is to be expected or found in every living human being. In principle, it is aristocratic.

---

*Additional linguistic evidence may enrich our inquiry. *Dignitas* means (1) a being worthy, worthiness, merit, desert; (2) dignity, greatness, grandeur, authority, rank; and (3) (of inanimate things) worth, value, excellence. The noun is cognate with the adjective *dignus*, "pointed out" or "shown," and hence, "worthy" or "deserving" (of persons), and "suitable," "fitting," "becoming," or "proper" (of things). "Dignity," in the *Oxford English Dictionary*, is said to have eight meanings; the four relevant ones I reproduce here: (1) The quality of being worthy or honourable; worthiness, worth, nobleness, excellence (for instance, "The real dignity of a man lies not in what he has, but in what he is," or "The dignity of this act was worth the audience of kings"); (2) Honourable or high estate, position, or estimation; honour, degrees of estimation, rank (for instance, "Stones, though in dignitie of nature inferior to plants," or "Clay and clay differs in dignity, whose dust is both alike"); (3) An honourable office, rank, or title; a high official or titular position (for instance, "He ... distributed the civil and military dignities among his favorites and followers"); (4) Nobility or befitting elevation of aspect, manner, or style; becoming or fit stateliness, gravity (for instance, "A dignity of dress adorns the Great").

It follows that dignity, thus understood, cannot be demanded or claimed; for it cannot be provided and it is not owed. One has no more *right* to dignity—and hence to dignity in death—than one has to beauty or courage or wisdom, desirable though these may be.

One can, of course, seek to democratize the principle; one can argue that "excellence," "being worthy" is a property of all human beings, for example, in comparison with animals or plants or machines. This, I take it, is what is often meant by *"human* dignity." This is also what is implied when it is asserted that much of the terminal treatment of dying patients is dehumanizing, or that attachments to catheters, respirators and suction tubes hide the human countenance and thereby insult the dignity of the dying. I myself earlier argued that the special dignity of the human species, thus understood, is the ground of the sanctity of human life. Yet on further examination this universal attribution of dignity to human beings pays tribute more to human potentiality, to the *possibilities* for human excellence. *Full* dignity, or dignity properly so-called, would depend on the *realization* of these possibilities.

Moreover, to speak of dignity as predicable of all human beings in contrast to animals, for instance, is once again to tie dignity to those distinctively human features of human animals, such as thought, image making, the sense of beauty, freedom, friendship, and the moral life, and not the mere presence of life itself. Among human beings, there would still be, on any such material principle, distinctions to be made. If universal human dignity is grounded, for example, in the moral life, in that everyone faces and makes moral choices, dignity would seem to depend mainly on having a *good* moral life, that is, on choosing well. Is there not more dignity in the courageous than in the cowardly, in the moderate than in the self-indulgent, in the righteous than in the wicked?*

But courage, moderation, righteousness and the other human virtues are not solely confined to the few. Many of us strive for them,

---

*This is not necessarily to say that one should treat other people, including those who eschew dignity, as if they lacked it. This is a separable question. It may be salutary to treat people on the basis of their capacities to live humanly, despite even great falling short or willful self-degradation. Yet this would, in the moral sphere at least, require that we expect and demand of people that they behave worthily and that we hold them responsible for their own conduct.

with partial success, and still more of us do ourselves honor when we recognize and admire those people nobler and finer than ourselves. With proper models, proper rearing and proper encouragement, many of us can be and act more in accord with our higher natures. In these ways, the openness to dignity can perhaps be democratized still further.

In truth, if we know how to look, we find evidence of human dignity all around us, in the valiant efforts ordinary people make to meet necessity, to combat adversity and disappointment, to provide for their children, to care for their parents, to help their neighbors, to serve their country. Life provides numerous hard occasions that call for endurance and equanimity, generosity and kindness, courage and self-command. Adversity sometimes brings out the best in a man, and often shows best what he is made of. Confronting our own death—or the deaths of our beloved ones—provides an opportunity for the exercise of our humanity, for the great and small alike. Death with dignity, in its most important sense, would mean a dignified attitude and virtuous conduct in the face of death.

What would such a dignified facing of death require? First of all, it would require knowing that one is dying. One cannot attempt to settle accounts, make arrangements, complete projects, keep promises or say farewell if one does not know the score. Second, it requires that one remain to some degree an agent rather than (just) a patient. One cannot make a good end of one's life if one is buffeted about by forces beyond one's control, if one is denied a decisive share in decisions about medical treatments, institutionalization, and the way to spend one's remaining time. Third, it requires the upkeep—as much as possible—of one's familial, social and professional relationships and activities. One cannot function as an actor if one has been swept off the stage and been abandoned by the rest of the cast. It would also seem to require some direct, self-conscious confrontation, in the loneliness of one's soul, with the brute fact and meaning of nearing one's end. Even, or especially, as he must be passive to the forces of decay, the dignified human being can preserve and reaffirm his humanity by seeing clearly and without illusion.* (It is for this reason, among

---

*The Homeric warriors, preoccupied with mortality and refusing to hide away in a corner waiting for death to catch them unawares, went boldly forward to meet it,

others, that sudden and unexpected death, however painless, robs a man of the opportunity to have a dignified end.)

But as a dignified human life is not just a lonely project against an inevitable death, but a life whose meaning is entwined in human relationships, we must stress again the importance for a death with dignity—as for a life with dignity—of dignified human intercourse with all those around us. Who we are to ourselves is largely inseparable from who we are to and for others; thus, our own exercise of dignified humanity will depend crucially on continuing to receive respectful treatment from others. The manner in which we are addressed, what is said to us or in our presence, how our bodies are tended or our feelings regarded—in all these ways, our dignity in dying can be nourished and sustained. Dying people are all too easily reduced ahead of time to "thinghood" by those who cannot bear to deal with the suffering or disability of those they love. Objectification and detachment are understandable defenses. Yet this withdrawal of contact, affection and care is probably the greatest single cause of the dehumanization of dying. Death with dignity requires absolutely that the survivors treat the human being at all times as if full godlikeness remains, up to the very end.

It will, I hope, now be perfectly clear that death with dignity, understood as living dignifiedly in the face of death, is not a matter of pulling plugs or taking poison. To speak this way—and it is unfortunately common to speak this way*—is to shrink still further the notion of human dignity, and thus heap still greater indignity upon the dying, beyond all the insults of illness and the medicalized bureaucratization of the end of life. If it really is death with dignity we are after, we must think in human and not technical terms. With these

---

armed only with their own prowess and large hearts; in facing death frontally, in the person of another similarly self-conscious hero, they wrested a human victory over blind necessity, even in defeat. On a much humbler scale, the same opportunity is open to anyone willing to look death in the face.

*A perfect instance, some years back, was a California initiative that sought to change the name of an existing California statute from "Natural Death Act" to "Humane and Dignified Death Act." Its only substantive change was to declare and provide for "the right of the terminally ill to voluntary, humane, and dignified doctor-assisted aid in dying," "aid in dying" meaning "any medical procedure that will terminate the life of the qualified patient swiftly, painlessly, and humanely." A (merely) natural death is to be made "dignified" simply by having it deliberately produced by (dignified) doctors.

thoughts firmly in mind, we can turn in closing back to the matter of euthanasia.

## Euthanasia: Undignified and Dangerous

Having followed the argument to this point, even a friendly reader might chide me as follows: "Well and good to think humanistically, but tough practical dilemmas arise, precisely about the use of techniques, and they must be addressed. Not everyone is so fortunate as to be able to die at home, in the company of loving family, beyond the long reach of the medical-industrial complex. How should these technical decisions—about respirators and antibiotics and feeding tubes and, yes, even poison—be made, precisely in order to uphold human dignity and the sanctity of life that you say are so intermingled?" A fair question. I offer the following outline of an answer.

About treatment for the actually dying, there is in principle no difficulty. Elsewhere I have argued for the primacy of easing pain and suffering, along with supporting and comforting speech, and, more to the point, the need to draw back from some efforts at prolongation of life that prolong or increase only the patient's pain, discomfort and suffering. Although I am mindful of the dangers and aware of the impossibility of writing explicit rules for easing treatment—hence the need for prudence—considerations of the individual's health, activity and state of mind must enter into decisions of *whether* and *how vigorously* to treat if the decision is indeed to be for the patient's good. Ceasing treatment and allowing death to occur when (and if) it will, can, under some circumstances, be quite compatible with the respect that life itself commands for itself. For life can be revered not only in its preservation, but also in the manner in which we allow a given life to reach its terminus.

What about so-called active euthanasia, the direct making dead of someone who is not yet dying or not dying "fast enough"? Elsewhere I have argued at great length against the practice of euthanasia *by physicians,* partly on the grounds of bad social consequences, but mainly on the grounds that killing patients—even those who ask for death—violates the inner meaning of the art of healing.[1] Powerful prudential arguments—unanswerable, in my view—have been advanced as to why legalized mercy killing would be a disastrous social policy, at least for the United States. But some will insist that social policy cannot remain deaf to cries for human dignity, and that dangers must be run to preserve a dignified death through euthanasia, at least where it is requested. As our theme here is dignity and sanctity, I will confine my answer to the question of euthanasia and human dignity.

Let us begin with voluntary euthanasia—the request for assistance in dying. To repeat, the claim here is that the choice for death, because a free act, affirms the dignity of free will against dumb necessity. Or, using my earlier formulation, is it not precisely dignified for the "godlike" to put a voluntary end to the humiliation of that very godliness?

In response, let me start with the following questions. Do the people who are actually contemplating euthanasia *for themselves*—as opposed to their proxies who lead the euthanasia movement—generally put their requests in these terms? Or are they not rather looking for a way to end their troubles and pains? One can sympathize with such a motive, out of compassion, but can one admire it, out of respect? Is it really dignified to seek to escape from troubles for oneself? Is there, to repeat, not more dignity in courage than in its absence?

Euthanasia for one's own dignity is, at best, paradoxical, even self-contradictory: how can I honor myself by making myself nothing? Even if dignity were to consist solely in autonomy, is it not an embarrassment to claim that autonomy reaches its zenith precisely as it disappears? Voluntary euthanasia, in the name of *positive* dignity, does not make sense.

Acknowledging the paradox, some will still argue the cause of freedom on a narrower ground: the prospect of euthanasia increases human freedom by increasing options. It is, of course, a long theoretical question whether human freedom is best understood—and best served—through the increase of possibilities. But as a practical matter, in the present case, I am certain that this view is mistaken. On the contrary, the opening up of this "option" of assisted suicide will greatly constrain human choice. For the choice for death is not one option among many, but an option to end all options. Socially, there will be great pressure on the aged and the vulnerable to exercise this option. Once there looms the legal alternative of euthanasia, it will plague and burden every decision made by any seriously ill elderly person—not to speak of their more powerful caretakers—even without the subtle hints and pressures applied to them by others.

And, thinking about others, is it dignified to ask or demand that someone else become my killer? It may be sad that one is unable to end one's own life, but can it conduce to either party's dignity to make the request? Consider its double meaning if made to a son or daughter: Do you love me so little as to force me to live on? Do you love me so little as to want me dead? What person in full possession of their own dignity would inflict such a duty on anyone they loved?

Of course, the whole thing could be made impersonal. No requests to family members, only to physicians. But precisely the same point applies: how can one demand care and humanity from one's physician, and, at the same time, demand that he play the role of technical dispenser of death? To turn the matter over to non-physicians, that is, to technically competent professional euthanizers, is, of course, to completely dehumanize the matter.*

Proponents of euthanasia do not understand human dignity, which, at best, they confuse with humaneness. One of their favorite arguments proves this point: why, they say, do we put animals out of their misery but insist on compelling fellow human beings to suffer to the bitter end? Why, if it is not a contradiction for the veterinarian, does the medical ethic absolutely rule out mercy killing? Is this not simply inhumane?

Perhaps inhumane, but not thereby inhuman. On the contrary, it is precisely because animals are not human that we must treat them (merely) humanely. We put dumb animals to sleep because they do not know that they are dying, because they can make nothing of their misery or mortality, and because, therefore, they cannot live deliberately—that is, humanly—in the face of their own suffering or dying. They cannot live out a fitting end. Compassion for

---

*For a chilling picture of the fully rationalized and technically managed death, see the account of the Park Lane Hospital for the Dying in Aldous Huxley's *Brave New World*.

their weakness and dumbness is our only appropriate emotion, and given our responsibility for their care and well-being, we do the only humane thing we can. But when a conscious human being asks us for death, by that very action he displays the presence of something that precludes our regarding him as a dumb animal. Humanity is owed humanity, not humaneness. Humanity is owed the bolstering of the human, even or especially in its dying moments, in resistance to the temptation to ignore its presence in the sight of suffering.

What humanity needs most in the face of evils is courage, the ability to stand against fear and pain and thoughts of nothingness. The deaths we most admire are those of people who, knowing that they are dying, face the fact frontally and act accordingly: they set their affairs in order, they arrange what could be final meetings with their loved ones, and yet, with strength of soul and a small reservoir of hope, they continue to live and work and love as much as they can for as long as they can. Because such conclusions of life require courage, they call for our encouragement—and for the many small speeches and deeds that shore up the human spirit against despair and defeat.

And what of nonvoluntary euthanasia, for those too disabled to request it for themselves—the comatose, the senile, the psychotic: can this be said to be in the service of *their* human dignity? If dignity is, as the autonomy people say, tied crucially to consciousness and will, nonvoluntary or "proxy-voluntary" euthanasia can never be a dignified act for the one euthanized. Indeed, it is precisely the absence of dignified humanity that invites the thought of active euthanasia in the first place.

Is it really true that such people are beneath all human dignity? I suppose it depends on the particulars. Many people in greatly reduced states still retain clear, even if partial, participation in human relations. They may respond to kind words or familiar music; they may keep up pride in their appearance or in the achievements of the grandchildren; they may take pleasure in reminiscences or simply in having someone who cares enough to be present; conversely, they may be irritated or hurt or sad, even appropriately so; and, even nearer bottom, they may be able to return a smile or a glance in response to a drink of water or a change of bedding or a bath. Because we really do not know their inner life—what they feel and understand—we run the risk of robbing them of opportunities for dignity by treating them as if they had none. It does not follow from the fact that *we* would never willingly trade places with them that *they* have nothing left worth respecting.

But what, finally, about the very bottom of the line, say, people in a "persistent vegetative state," unresponsive, contorted, with no evident ability to interact with the environment? What human dignity remains here? Why should we not treat such human beings as we (properly) treat dumb animals, and put them out of "their misery"?* I grant that one faces here the hardest case for the argument I am advancing. Yet one probably cannot be absolutely sure, even here, about the complete absence of inner life or awareness of their surroundings. In some cases, admittedly extremely rare, persons recover from profound coma; and they sometimes report having had partial yet vivid awareness of what was said and done to them, though they had given no external evidence of same. But beyond any restraint owing to ignorance, I would also myself be restrained by the human form, by *human blood,* and by what I owe to the full human life that this particular instance of humanity once lived. I would gladly stand aside and let die, say in the advent of pneumonia; I would do little beyond the minimum to sustain life; but I would not countenance the giving of lethal injections or the taking of other actions deliberately intending the patient's death. Between only undignified courses of action, this strikes me as the least undignified—especially for myself.

I have no illusions that it is easy to live with a Karen Ann Quinlan or a Nancy Cruzan. I think I sufficiently appreciate the anguish of their parents or their children, and the distortion of their lives and the lives of their families. I also know that when hearts break and people can stand it no longer, mercy killing will happen, and I

---

*Once again we should be careful about our speech. It may be a great source of misery for us to see them in this state, but it is not at all clear that *they feel* or *have* misery. Precisely the ground for considering them beneath the human threshold is that *nothing* registers with them. This point is relevant to the "termination-of-feeding" cases, in which it is argued (in self-contradiction) that death by starvation is both humane and not in these instances cruel: someone who is too far gone to suffer from death by starvation is, to begin with, not suffering at all.

think we should be prepared to excuse it—as we generally do—when it occurs in this way. But an excuse is not yet a justification, and very far from dignity.

What then should we conclude, as a matter of social policy? We should reject the counsel of those who, seeking to drive a wedge between human dignity and the sanctity of life, argue the need for active euthanasia, especially in the name of death with dignity. For it is precisely the setting of fixed limits on violating human life that makes possible our efforts at dignified relations with our fellow men, especially when their neediness and disability try our patience. We will never be able to relate even decently to people if we are entitled always to consider that one option before us is to make them dead. Thus, when the advocates for euthanasia press us with the most heartrending cases, we should be sympathetic but firm. Our response should be neither "Yes, for mercy's sake" nor "Murder! Unthinkable!" but "Sorry. No." Above all we must not allow ourselves to become self-deceived: we must never seek to relieve *our own* frustrations and bitterness over the lingering deaths of others by pretending that we can kill them to sustain *their dignity.*

The ancient Greeks knew about hubris and its tragic fate. We modern rationalists do not. We do not yet understand that the project for the conquest of death leads only to dehumanization, that any attempt to regain the tree of eternal life by means of the tree of knowledge leads inevitably also to the hemlock, and that the utter rationalization of life under the banner of the will gives rise to a world in which the victors would live long enough to finish life demented and without choice. The human curse is to discover only too late the evils latent in acquiring the goods we wish for.

Against the background of enormous medical success, terminal illness and incurable disease appear as failures and as affronts to human pride. We refuse to be caught resourceless. Thus, having adopted a largely technical approach to human life and having medicalized so much of the end of life, we now are willing to contemplate a final technical solution for the evil of human finitude and for our own technical (but unavoidable) "failure," as well as for the degradations of life that are the unintended consequences of our technical successes. This is dangerous folly. People who care for autonomy and human dignity should try rather to reverse this dehumanization of the last stages of life, instead of giving dehumanization its final triumph by welcoming the desperate goodbye-to-all-that contained in one final plea for poison.

The present crisis that leads some to press for assisted suicide and active euthanasia is really an opportunity to learn the limits of the medicalization of life and death and to recover an appreciation of living with and against mortality. It is an opportunity to remember and affirm that there remains a residual human wholeness— however precarious—that can be cared for even in the face of incurable and terminal illness. Should we cave in, should we choose to become technical dispensers of death, we will not only be abandoning our loved ones and our duty to care; we will exacerbate the worst tendencies of modern life, embracing technicism and "humaneness" where encouragement and humanity are both required and sorely lacking. On the other hand, should we hold fast, should we decline the "ethics of choice" and its deadly options, should we learn that finitude is no disgrace and that human dignity can be cared for to the very end, we may yet be able to stem the rising tide that threatens permanently to submerge the best hopes for human dignity.

# CHAPTER NINE

# L'Chaim *and Its Limits:*
# *Why Not Immortality?*

You don't have to be Jewish to drink *L'Chaim*, to lift a glass "To Life." Everyone in his right mind believes that life is good and death is bad. But Jews have always had an unusually keen appreciation of life, and not only because it has been stolen from them so often and so cruelly. The celebration of life—of *this* life, not the next one—has from the beginning been central to Jewish ethical and religious sensibilities. In the Torah, "Be fruitful and multiply" is God's first blessing and first command. Judaism from its inception rejected child sacrifice and regarded long life as a fitting divine reward for righteous living. At the same time, Judaism embraces medicine and the human activity of healing the sick; from the Torah the rabbis deduced not only permission for doctors to heal, but also the positive obligation to do so. Indeed, so strong is this reverence for life that the duty of *pikuah nefesh* requires that Jews violate the holy Shabbat in order to save a life. Not by accident do we Jews raise our glasses *L'Chaim*.

Neither is it accidental that Jews have been enthusiastic boosters of modern medicine and biomedical science. Vastly out of proportion to their numbers, they build hospitals and laboratories, support medical research, and see their sons and daughters in the vanguard wherever new scientific discoveries are to be made and new remedies to be found. Yet this beloved biomedical project, for all its blessings, now raises for Jews and for all humanity a plethora of serious and often unprecedented moral challenges. Laboratory-assisted reproduction, artificial organs, genetic manipulation, psychoactive drugs, computer implants in the brain, techniques to conquer aging—these and other present and projected techniques for altering our bodies and minds pose challenges to the very meaning of our humanity. Our growing power to control human life may require us to consider possible limits to the principle of *L'Chaim*.

One well-known set of challenges results from undesired consequences of medical success in sustaining life, as more and more people are kept alive by artificial means in greatly debilitated and degraded conditions. When, if ever, is it permissible for doctors to withhold antibiotics, discontinue a respirator, remove a feeding tube, or even assist in suicide or perform euthanasia?

A second set of challenges concerns the morality of means used to seek the cure of disease or the creation of life. Is it ethical to create living human embryos for the sole purpose of experimenting on them? To conceive a child in order that it may become a compatible bone marrow donor for an afflicted sibling? Is it ethical to practice human cloning to provide a child for an infertile couple?

Third, we may soon face challenges concerning the goal itself: Should we, partisans of life, welcome efforts to increase not just the average but also the *maximum* human lifespan, by attempting to conquer aging, decay, and ultimately mortality itself?

In the debates taking place in the United States, Jewish commentators on these and related topics in medical ethics nearly always come down strongly in favor of medical progress and on the side of life—more life, longer life, new life. They treat the cure of disease, the prevention of death and the extension of life as near-absolute values, trumping most if not all other moral objections. Unlike, say, Roman Catholic moralists who hold to certain natural law teachings that set limits on permissible practice, the Jewish commentators, even if they acknowledge difficulties, ultimately wind up saying that life and health are good, and that therefore whatever serves more of each and both is better.

Let me give two examples out of my own experience. Five years ago, when I gave testimony on the ethics of human cloning before the National Bioethics Advisory Commission, I was surprised to discover that the two experts who had been invited to testify on the Jewish point of view were not especially troubled by the prospect. The Orthodox rabbi, invoking the goodness of life and the injunction to be fruitful and multiply, held that cloning of the husband or the wife to provide a child for an infertile couple was utterly unobjectionable according to Jewish law. The Conservative rabbi, while acknowledging certain worries, concluded: "If cloning human beings is intended to advance medical research or cure infertility, it has a proper place in God's scheme of things, understood in the Jewish tradition." Let someone else worry about Brave-New-Worldly turning procreation into manufacture or the meaning of replacing heterosexual procreation by asexual propagation. Prospective cures for diseases and children for infertile couples suffice to legitimate human cloning—and, by extension, will legitimate farming human embryos for spare body parts or even creating babies in bottles when that becomes feasible.

The second example: At a meeting in March 2000 on "Extended Life, Eternal Life," scientists and theologians were invited to discuss the desirability of increasing the maximum human lifespan to, say, 150 years and, more radically, of treating death itself as a disease to be conquered. The major Jewish speaker, a professor at a leading rabbinical seminary, embraced the project—you should excuse me—whole hog. Gently needling his Christian colleagues by asserting that for Jews, God is Life rather than Love, he used this principle to justify any and all life-preserving and life-extending technologies, including those that might yield massive increases in the maximum human life expectancy. When I pressed him in discussion to see if he had any objections to the biomedical pursuit of immortality, he responded that Judaism would only welcome such a project.

I am prepared to accept the view that traditional Jewish sources may be silent on these matters, given that the *halakhah* could know nothing about test-tube babies, cloning or the campaign to conquer aging. But in my opinion, such unqualified endorsement of medical progress and the unlimited pursuit of longevity cannot be the counsel of wisdom, and therefore, should not be the counsel of Jewish wisdom. *L'Chaim,* I say, but with limits.

Let us address the question of *L'Chaim* and its limits in its starkest and most radical form: If life is good and more is better, should we not regard death as a disease and try to cure it? Although this formulation of the question may seem too futuristic or far-fetched, there are several reasons for taking it up and treating it seriously.

First, reputable scientists are today answering the question in the affirmative and are already making large efforts toward bringing about a cure. Three kinds of research, still in their infancy, are attracting new attention and energies. First is the use of hormones, especially human growth hormone (hGH), to restore and enhance youthful bodily vigor. In the United States, over ten thousand people—including many physicians—are already injecting themselves daily with hGH for anti-aging purposes, with apparently remarkable improvements in bodily fitness and performance, though there is as yet no evidence that the hormones yield any increase in life expectancy. When the patent on hGH expires in 2002 and the cost comes down from its current $1,000 per month, many more people are almost certainly going to be injecting themselves from the hormonal fountain of youth.

Second is research on stem cells, those omnicompetent primordial cells that, on different signals, turn into all the various differentiated tissues of the body—liver, heart, kidney, brain and so on. Stem cell technologies hold out the promise of an indefinite supply of replacement tissues and organs for any and all worn-out body parts. This is a booming area in commercial biotechnology, and one of the leading biotech entrepreneurs has been touting his company's research as promising indefinite prolongation of life.

Third, there is research into the genetic switches that control the biological processes of aging. The maximum lifespan for each species—roughly one hundred years for human beings—is almost certainly under genetic control. In a startling recent discovery, fruit-fly geneticists have shown that mutations in a single gene produce a 50 percent increase in the natural lifetime of the flies. Once the genes involved in regulating the human life cycle and setting the midnight hour are identified, scientists predict that they will be able to increase the human maximum age well beyond its natural limit. Quite frankly, I find some of the claims and predictions to be overblown, but it would be foolhardy to bet against scientific and technical progress along these lines.

Yet even if cures for aging and death are a long way off, there is a second and more fundamental reason for inquiring into the radical question of the desirability of gaining a cure for death. For truth to tell, victory over mortality is the unstated but implicit goal of modern medical science, indeed of the entire modern scientific project, to which mankind was summoned almost four hundred years ago by Francis Bacon and René Descartes. They quite consciously trumpeted the conquest of nature for the relief of man's estate, and they founded a science whose explicit purpose was to reverse the curse laid on Adam and Eve, and especially to restore the tree of life, by means of the tree of (scientific) knowledge. With medicine's increasing successes, realized mainly in the last half-century, every death is increasingly regarded as premature, a failure of today's medicine that future research will prevent. In parallel with medical progress, a new moral sensibility has developed that serves precisely medicine's crusade against mortality: anything is permitted if it saves life, cures disease, prevents death. Regardless, therefore, of the imminence of anti-aging remedies, it is most worthwhile to reexamine the assumption upon which we have been operating: that everything should be done to preserve health and prolong life as much as possible, and that all other values must bow before the biomedical gods of better health, greater vigor and longer life.

Recent proposals that we should conquer aging and death have not been without their critics. The criticism takes two forms: predictions of bad social consequences and complaints about distributive justice. Regarding the former, there are concerns about the effect on the size and age distribution of the population. How will growing numbers and percentages of people living well past one hundred affect, for example, work opportunities, retirement plans, hiring and promotion, cultural attitudes and beliefs, the structure of family life, relations between the generations, or the locus of rule and authority in government, business and the professions? Even the most cursory examination of these matters suggests that the cumulative results of aggregated decisions for longer and more vigorous life could be highly disruptive and undesirable, even to the point that many individuals would be *worse off* through most of their lives, and enough to offset the benefits of better health afforded them near the end of life. Indeed, several people have predicted that retardation of aging will present a classic instance of the "Tragedy of the Commons," in which genuine and sought-for gains to individuals are nullified, or worse, by the social consequences of granting them to everyone.

But other critics worry that technology's gift of long or immortal life will not be granted to everyone, especially if, as is likely, the treatments turn out to be expensive. Would it not be the ultimate injustice if only some people could afford a deathless existence, if the world were divided not only into rich and poor but into mortal and immortal?

Against these critics, the proponents of immortality research answer confidently that we will gradually figure out a way to solve these problems. We can handle any adverse social consequences through careful planning; we can overcome the inequities through cheaper technologies. Though I think these optimists woefully naive, let me for the moment grant their view regarding these issues. For both the proponents and their critics have yet to address thoughtfully the heart of the matter, the question of the goodness of the goal. The core question is this: Is it really true that longer life for individuals is an unqualified good?

## The Proper Lifespan

How *much* longer life is a blessing for an individual? Ignoring now the possible harms flowing back to individuals from adverse social consequences, how much more life is good for us as individuals, other things being equal? How much more life do we want, assuming it to be healthy and vigorous? Assuming that it were up to us to set the human lifespan, where would or should we set the limit and why?

The simple answer is that no limit should be set. Life is good and death is bad. Therefore, the more life the better, provided, of course, that we remain fit and our friends do, too.

This answer has the virtues of clarity and honesty. But most public advocates of conquering aging deny any such greediness. They hope not for immortality, but for something reasonable—just a few more years.

How many years are reasonably few? Let us start with ten. Which of us would find unreasonable or unwelcome the addition of ten healthy and vigorous years to his or her life, years like those between ages thirty and forty? We could learn more, earn more, see more, do more. Maybe we should ask for five years on top of that? Or ten? Why not fifteen, or twenty, or more?

If we can't immediately land on the reasonable number of added years, perhaps we can locate the principle. What is the principle of reasonableness? Time needed for our plans and projects yet to be completed? Some multiple of the age of a generation, say, that we might live to see great-grandchildren fully grown? Some notion—traditional, natural, revealed—of the proper lifespan for a being such as man? We have no answer to this question. We do not even know how to choose among the principles for setting our new lifespan.

Under such circumstances, lacking a standard of reasonableness, we fall back on our wants and desires. Under liberal democracy, this means the desires of the majority for whom the attachment to life—or the fear of death—knows no limits. It turns out that the simple answer is the best: we want to live and live, not to wither and die. For most of us, especially under modern secular conditions in which more and more people believe that this is the only life they have, the desire to prolong the lifespan (even modestly) must be seen as expressing a desire never to grow old and die. However naive their counsel, those who propose immortality deserve credit: they honestly and shamelessly expose this desire.

Some, of course, eschew any desire for longer life. They seek not adding years to life, but life to years. For them, the ideal lifespan would be our natural (once thought threescore and ten, now known to be) fourscore and ten, or if by reason of strength, fivescore, lived with full powers right up to death, which could come rather suddenly, painlessly, at the maximal age. This has much to recommend it. Who would not want to avoid senility, crippling arthritis, the need for hearing aids and dentures, and the degrading dependencies of old age? But in the absence of these degenerations, would we remain content to spurn longer life? Would we not become even more disinclined to exit? Would not death become even more of an affront? Would not the fear and loathing of death increase in the absence of its harbingers? We could no longer comfort the widow by pointing out that her husband was delivered from his suffering. Death would always be untimely, unprepared for, shocking.

Montaigne saw it clearly:

> I notice that in proportion as I sink into sickness, I naturally enter into a certain disdain for life. I find that I have much

more trouble digesting this resolution when I am in health than when I have a fever. Inasmuch as I no longer cling so hard to the good things of life when I begin to lose the use and pleasure of them, I come to view death with much less frightened eyes. This makes me hope that the farther I get from life and the nearer to death, the more easily I shall accept the exchange.... If we fell into such a change [decrepitude] suddenly, I don't think we could endure it. But when we are led by Nature's hand down a gentle and virtually imperceptible slope, bit by bit, one step at a time, she rolls us into this wretched state and makes us familiar with it; so that we find no shock when youth dies within us, which in essence and in truth is a harder death than the complete death of a languishing life or the death of old age; inasmuch as the leap is not so cruel from a painful life as from a sweet and flourishing life to a grievous and painful one.

Thus it is highly likely that even a modest prolongation of life with vigor or even only a preservation of youthfulness with no increase in longevity would make death less acceptable and would exacerbate the desire to keep pushing it away—unless, for some reason, such life could also prove less satisfying.

Could longer, healthier life be less satisfying? How could it be, if life is good and death is bad? Perhaps the simple view is in error. Perhaps mortality is not simply an evil, perhaps it is even a blessing—not only for the welfare of the community, but even for us as individuals. How could this be?

I wish to make the case for the virtues of mortality. Against my own strong love of life, and against my even stronger wish that no more of my loved ones should die, I aspire to speak truth to my desires by showing that the finitude of human life is a blessing for every human individual, whether he knows it or not.

I know I won't persuade many people to my position. But I do hope I can convince readers of the gravity—I would say, the unique gravity—of this question. We are not talking about some minor new innovation with ethical wrinkles about which we may chatter or regulate as usual. Conquering death is not something that we can try for a while and then decide whether the results are better or worse—according to, God only knows, what standard. On the contrary, this is a question in which our very humanity is at stake, not only in the consequences but also in the very meaning of the choice. For to argue that human life would be better without death is, I submit, to argue that human life would be better being something other than human. To be immortal would not be just to continue life as we mortals now know it, only forever. The new immortals, in the decisive sense, would not be like us at all. If this is true, a human choice for bodily immortality would suffer from the deep confusion of choosing to have some great good only on the condition of turning into someone else. Moreover, such an immortal someone else, in my view, will be less well off than we mortals are now, thanks indeed to our mortality.

## The Virtues of Mortality

It goes without saying that there is no virtue in the death of a child or a young adult, or the untimely or premature death of anyone, before they had attained to the measure of man's days. Neither am I suggesting that there is virtue in the particular *event* of death for anyone or that separation through death is anything but painful for the survivors, those for whom the deceased was an integral part of their lives. Instead, my question concerns the fact of our finitude, the fact of our mortality—the fact *that we must die,* the fact that a full life for a human being has a biological, built-in limit, one that has evolved as part of our nature. Does this fact also have value? Is our finitude good for us—as individuals? (I intend this question entirely in the realm of natural reason and apart from any question about a life after death.)

To praise mortality must seem to be madness. If mortality is a blessing, it surely is not widely regarded as such. Life seeks to live, and rightly suspects all counsels of finitude. "Better to be a slave on earth than the king over all the dead," says Achilles in Hades to the visiting Odysseus, in apparent regret for his prior choice of the short but glorious life. Moreover, though some cultures—such as the Eskimo—can instruct and moderate somewhat the lust for life, liberal Western society gives it free rein, beginning with a political philosophy founded on a fear of violent death, and reaching to our current cults of youth and novelty, the cosmetic replastering of the wrinkles of age, and the widespread anxiety about disease and survival. Finally, the virtues of finitude—if there are any—may never be widely appreciated in any age or culture, if appreciation depends on a certain wisdom, if wisdom requires a certain detachment from the love of oneself and one's own, and if the possibility of such detachment is given only to the few. Still, if it is wisdom, the rest of us should hearken, for we may learn something of value for ourselves.

How, then, might our finitude be good for us? I offer four benefits, first among which is *interest and engagement.* If the human lifespan were increased even by only twenty years, would the pleasures of life increase proportionally? Would professional tennis players really enjoy playing 25 percent more games of tennis? Would the Don Juans of our world feel better for having seduced 1,250 women rather than 1,000? Having experienced the joys and tribulations of raising a family until the last had left for college, how many parents would like to extend the experience by another ten years? Likewise, those whose satisfaction comes from climbing the career ladder might well ask what there would be to do for fifteen years after one had been CEO of Microsoft, a member of Congress, or the president of Harvard for a quarter of a century? Even less clear are the additions to personal happiness from more of the same of the less pleasant and less fulfilling activities in which so many of us are engaged so much of the time. It seems to be as the poet says: "We move and ever spend our lives amid the same things, and not by any length of life is any new pleasure hammered out."

Second, *seriousness and aspiration.* Could life be serious or meaningful without the limit of mortality? Is not the limit on our time the ground of our taking life seriously and living it passionately? To know and to feel that one goes around only once, and that the deadline is not out of sight, is for many people the necessary spur to the pursuit of something worthwhile. "Teach us to number our days," says the Psalmist, "that we may get a heart of wisdom." To number our days is the condition for making them count. Homer's immortals—Zeus and Hera, Apollo and Athena—for all their eternal beauty and youthfulness, live shallow and rather frivolous lives, their passions only transiently engaged, in first this and then that. They live as spectators of the mortals, who by comparison have depth, aspiration, genuine feeling, and hence a real center in their lives. Mortality makes life matter.

There may be some activities, especially in some human beings, that do not require finitude as a spur. A powerful desire for understanding can do without external proddings, let alone one related to mortality; and as there is never too much time to learn and to understand, longer, more vigorous life might be simply a boon. The best sorts of friendship, too, seem capable of indefinite growth, especially where growth is somehow tied to learning—though one may wonder whether real friendship doesn't depend in part on the shared perceptions of a common fate. But, in any case, I suspect that these are among the rare exceptions. For most activities, and for most of us, I think it is crucial that we recognize and feel the force of not having world enough and time.

A third matter, *beauty and love.* Death, says the poet, is the mother of beauty. What he means is not easy to say. Perhaps he means that only a mortal being, aware of his mortality and the transience and vulnerability of all natural things, is moved to make beautiful artifacts, objects that will last, objects whose order will be immune to decay as their maker is not, beautiful objects that will bespeak and beautify a world that needs beautification, beautiful objects for other mortal beings who can appreciate what they cannot themselves make because of a taste for the beautiful, a taste perhaps connected to awareness of the ugliness of decay.

Perhaps the poet means to speak of natural beauty as well, which beauty—unlike that of objects of art—depends on its *im*permanence. Could the beauty of flowers depend on the fact that they will soon wither? Does the beauty of spring warblers depend upon the fall drabness that precedes and follows? What about the fading, late afternoon winter light or the spreading sunset? Is the beautiful necessarily fleeting, a peak that cannot be sustained? Or does the poet mean not that the beautiful is beautiful because mortal, but that our appreciation of its beauty depends on our appreciation of mortality—in us and in the beautiful? Does not love swell before the beautiful precisely on recognizing that it (and we) will not always be? Is not our mortality the cause of our enhanced appreciation of the beautiful and the worthy and of our treasuring and loving them? How deeply could one deathless "human" being love another?

Fourth, there is the peculiarly human beauty of character, *virtue and moral excellence.* To be mortal means that it is possible to give one's life, not only in one moment, say, on the field of battle, but also in the many other ways in which we are able in action to rise above attachment to survival. Through moral courage, endurance, greatness of soul, generosity, devotion to justice—in acts great and small—we rise above our mere creatureliness, spending the precious coinage of the time of our lives for the sake of the noble and the good and the holy. We free ourselves from fear, from bodily pleasures, or from attachments to wealth—all largely connected with survival—and in doing virtuous deeds overcome the weight of our neediness; yet for this nobility, vulnerability and mortality are the necessary conditions. The immortals cannot be noble.

Of this, too, the poets teach. Odysseus, long suffering, has already heard the shade of Achilles' testimony in praise of life when he is offered immortal life by the nymph Calypso. She is a beautiful goddess, attractive, kind, yielding; she sings sweetly and weaves on a golden loom; her island is well-ordered and lovely, free of hardships and suffering. Says the poet, "Even a god who came into that place would have admired what he saw, the heart delighted within him." Yet Odysseus turns down the offer to be lord of her household and immortal:

> Goddess and queen, do not be angry with me. I myself know that all you say is true and that circumspect Penelope can never match the impression you make for beauty and stature. She is mortal after all, and you are immortal and ageless. But even so, what I want and all my days I pine for is to go back to my house and see that day of my homecoming. And if some god batters me far out on the wine-blue water, I will endure it, keeping a stubborn spirit inside me, for already I have suffered much and done much hard work on the waves and in the fighting.

To suffer, to endure, to trouble oneself for the sake of home, family, community and genuine friendship, is truly to live, and is the clear choice of this exemplary mortal. This choice is both the mark of his excellence and the basis for the visible display of his excellence in deeds noble and just. Immortality is a kind of oblivion—like death itself.*

---

*The name Calypso means "one who hides or conceals or covers over."

## Longings for Immortality

But, someone might reasonably object, if mortality is such a blessing, why do so few cultures recognize it as such? Why do so many
teach the promise of life after death, of something eternal, of something imperishable? This takes us to the heart of the matter.

What is the meaning of this concern with immortality? *Why*
do we human beings seek immortality? Why do we want to live
longer or forever? Is it really first and most because we do not want
to die, because we do not want to leave this embodied life on earth
or give up our earthly pastimes, because we want to see more and
do more? I do not think so. This may be what we say, but it is not
what we finally mean. Mortality as such is not our defect, nor bodily immortality our goal. Rather, mortality is at most a pointer, a
derivative manifestation, or an accompaniment of some deeper deficiency. The promise of immortality and eternity answers rather to
a deep truth about the human soul: the human soul yearns for, longs
for, aspires to some condition, some state, some goal toward which
our earthly activities are directed but which cannot be attained in
earthly life. Our soul's reach exceeds our grasp; it seeks more than
continuance; it reaches for something beyond us, something that for
the most part eludes us. Our distress with mortality is the derivative manifestation of the conflict between the transcendent longings
of the soul and the all-too-finite powers and fleshly concerns of the
body.

What is it that we lack and long for, but cannot reach? One
possibility is completion in another person. For example, Plato's
Aristophanes says we seek wholeness through complete and permanent bodily and psychic union with a unique human being whom
we love, our "missing other half." Plato's Socrates, in contrast, says
it is rather wholeness through wisdom, through comprehensive
knowledge of the beautiful truth about the whole, that which philosophy seeks but can never attain. Yet again, biblical religion says
we seek wholeness through dwelling in God's presence, love and
redemption—a restoration of innocent wholeheartedness lost in the
Garden of Eden. But, please note, these and many other such accounts
of human aspiration, despite their differences, all agree on this crucial

point: man longs not so much for deathlessness as for wholeness, wisdom, goodness and godliness—longings that cannot be satisfied fully in our embodied earthly life, the only life, by natural reason, we know we have. Hence the attractiveness of any prospect or promise of a different and thereby fulfilling life hereafter.

The decisive inference is clear: none of these longings can be answered by prolonging earthly life. Not even an unlimited amount of "more of the same" will satisfy our deepest aspirations.

If this is correct, there follows a decisive corollary regarding the battle against death. The human taste for immortality, for the imperishable and the eternal, is not a taste that the biomedical conquest of death could satisfy. We would still be incomplete; we would still lack wisdom; we would still lack God's presence and redemption. Mere continuance will not buy fulfillment. Worse, its pursuit threatens—already threatens—human happiness by distracting us from the goals toward which our souls naturally point. By diverting our aim, by misdirecting so much individual and social energy toward the goal of bodily immortality, we may seriously undermine our chances for living as well as we can and for satisfying to some extent, however incompletely, our deepest longings for what is best. The implication for human life is hardly nihilistic: once we acknowledge and accept our finitude, we can concern ourselves with living well, and care first and most for the *well-being* of our souls, and not so much for their mere existence.

## Perpetuation

But perhaps this is all a mistake. Perhaps there is no such longing of the soul. Perhaps there is no soul. Certainly modern science doesn't speak about the soul; neither does medicine or even our psychiatrists (whose name means "healer of the soul"). Perhaps we are just animals, complex ones to be sure, but animals nonetheless, content just to be here, frightened in the face of danger, avoiding pain, seeking pleasure.

Curiously, however, biology has its own view of our nature and its inclinations. Biology also teaches about transcendence, though it eschews talk about the soul. Biology has long shown us a feasible way to rise above our finitude and to participate in something permanent and eternal: I refer not to stem cells, but to procreation—the bearing of and caring for offspring, for the sake of which many animals risk and even sacrifice their lives. Indeed, in all higher animals, reproduction *as such* implies both the acceptance of the death of self and participation in its transcendence. The salmon, willingly swimming upstream to spawn and die, makes vivid this universal truth.

But man is natured for more than spawning. Human biology teaches how our life points beyond itself—to our offspring, to our community, to our species. Like the other animals, man is built for reproduction. More than the other animals, man is also built for sociality. And, alone among the animals, man is also built for culture—not only through capacities to transmit and receive skills and techniques, but also through capacities for shared beliefs, opinions, rituals, traditions. We are built with leanings toward, and capacities for, perpetuation. Is it not possible that aging and mortality are part of this construction, and that the rate of aging and the human lifespan have been selected for their usefulness to the task of perpetuation? Could not extending the human lifespan place a great strain on our nature, jeopardizing our project and depriving us of success? Interestingly, perpetuation is a goal that is attainable, a transcendence of self that is (largely) realizable. Here is a form of participating in the enduring that is open to us, without qualification—provided, that is, that we remain open to it.

Biological considerations aside, simply to covet a prolonged lifespan for ourselves is both a sign and a cause of our failure to open ourselves to procreation and to any higher purpose. It is probably no accident that it is a generation whose intelligentsia proclaim the death of God and the meaninglessness of life that embarks on life's indefinite prolongation and that seeks to cure the emptiness of life by extending it forever. For the desire to prolong youthfulness is not only a childish desire to eat one's life and keep it; it is also an expression of a childish and narcissistic wish incompatible with devotion to posterity. It seeks an endless present, isolated from anything truly eternal, and severed from any true continuity with past and future. It is in principle hostile to children, because children, those who come after, are those who will take one's place; *they* are life's answer to mortality, and their presence in one's house is a constant reminder that one no longer belongs to the frontier generation. One cannot pursue agelessness for oneself and remain faithful to the spirit and meaning of perpetuation.

In perpetuation, we send forth not just the seed of our bodies, but also the bearer of our hopes, our truths, and those of our tradition. If our children are to flower, we need to sow them well and nurture them, cultivate them in rich and wholesome soil, clothe them in fine and decent opinions and mores, and direct them toward the highest light, to grow straight and tall—that they may take our place as we took that of those who planted us and made way for us, so that in time they, too, may make way and plant. But if they are truly to flower, we must go to seed; we must wither and give ground.

Against these considerations, the clever ones will propose that if we could do away with death, we would do away with the need for posterity. But that is a self-serving and shallow answer, one that thinks of life and aging solely in terms of the state of the body. It ignores the psychological effects simply of the passage of time—of experiencing and learning about the way things are. After a while, no matter how healthy we are, no matter how respected and well placed we are socially, most of us cease to look upon the world with fresh eyes. Little surprises us, nothing shocks us, righteous indignation at injustice dies out. We have seen it all already, seen it all. We have often been deceived, we have made many mistakes of our own. Many of us become small-souled, having been humbled not by bodily decline or the loss of loved ones but by life itself. So our ambition also begins to flag, or at least our noblest ambitions. As we grow older, Aristotle already noted, we "aspire to nothing great and exalted and crave the mere necessities and comforts of existence." At some point, most of us turn and say to our intimates, Is this all there is? We settle, we accept our situation—if we are lucky enough to be able to accept it. In many ways, perhaps in the most profound ways, most of us go to sleep long before our deaths—and we might even do so earlier in life if death no longer spurred us to make something of ourselves.

In contrast, it is in the young where aspiration, hope, freshness, boldness and openness spring anew—even when they take the form of overturning our monuments. Immortality for oneself through children may be a delusion, but participating in the natural and eternal renewal of human possibility through children is not—not even in today's world.

For it still stands as it did when Homer made Glaukos say to Diomedes:

> As is the generation of leaves, so is that of humanity. The wind scatters the leaves to the ground, but the live timber burgeons with leaves again in the season of spring returning. So one generation of man will grow while another dies.

And yet it also still stands, as this very insight of Homer's itself reveals, that human beings are in another respect unlike the leaves; that the eternal renewal of human beings embraces also the eternally human possibility of learning and self-awareness; that we, too, here and now may participate with Homer, with Plato, with the Bible, yes, with Descartes and Bacon, in catching at least some glimpse of the enduring truths about nature, God and human affairs; and that we, too, may hand down and perpetuate this pursuit of wisdom and goodness to our children and our children's children. Children and their education, not growth hormone and perpetual organ replacement, are life's—and wisdom's—answer to mortality.

This ancient Homeric wisdom is, in fact, not so far from traditional Jewish wisdom. For although we believe that life is good and long life is better, we hold something higher than life itself to be best. We violate one *Shabbat* so that the person whose life is saved may observe many *Shabbatoth*. We are obliged to accept death rather than commit idolatry, murder or sexual outrage. Though we love life and drink *L'Chaim,* we have been taught of old to love wisdom and justice and godliness more; among Jews, at least until recently, teachers were more revered than doctors. Regarding immortality, God Himself declares—in the Garden of Eden story—that human beings, once they have attained the burdensome knowledge of good and bad, should not have access to the tree of life. Instead, they are to cleave to the Torah as a tree of life, a life-perfecting path to righteousness and holiness. Unlike the death-defying Egyptians, those ancient precursors of the quest for bodily immortality, the Children of Israel do not mummify or embalm their dead; we bury our ancestors but keep them alive in memory, and, accepting our mortality, we look forward to the next generation. Indeed, the mitzvah to be fruitful and multiply (the Bible's first positive commandment), when rightly understood, celebrates not the life we have and selfishly would cling to, but the life that replaces us.

Confronted with the growing moral challenges posed by biomedical technology, let us resist the siren song of the conquest of aging and death. Let us cleave to our ancient wisdom and lift our voices and properly toast *L'Chaim,* to life beyond our own, to the life of our grandchildren and their grandchildren. May they, God willing, know health and long life, but especially so that they may also know the pursuit of truth and righteousness and holiness. And may they hand down and perpetuate this pursuit of what is humanly finest to succeeding generations for all time to come.

## ❋ Nature and
## Purposes of Biology

# CHAPTER TEN

# The Permanent Limitations of Biology

How far can biology take us? Are there limits on what it can know or on what it may enable us to do? According to many a prophet in the temple of science, biology has no permanent limitations. Instead, it faces an endless frontier—eagerly, gladly, confidently. Firmly founded on the concepts and methods of objective science, supported by the century-old doctrine of evolution, and armed with new discoveries and techniques in biochemistry and molecular genetics, biology and medicine go forward into a golden age. They promise, among other things, a full understanding of those age-old "mysteries" of embryogenesis and differentiation; an unlocking of the "secrets" of perception, memory, imagination and desire; new biotechnologies and new cures for disease; the provision of psychic peace through a true psychophysics; and perhaps even the conquest of mortality through mastery of the genetically determined processes of aging.

Not being a prophet myself, I cannot dispute these claims; indeed, I am rather inclined to believe them. But there is another meaning to the question of "permanent limitations," something quite independent of future events: Does biology have limitations that properly could be called permanent because they are intrinsic or inherent, unavoidably imbedded in the idea and practice of biology as such, regardless of how much more it comes to know? Are there activities of life, living things, or human living things that biology, *in principle,* cannot come to understand?

The answer depends in part on what we mean by "biology." What is biology? Is it primarily a kind of knowledge or a kind of power? If knowledge, knowledge of what? Of living things, or of "life," or of vital processes? Of what things *are,* or of how they *work?* If power, power to do what, to whom, and why? Power to predict and control, or power to cure disease and prolong life, or power to do and to make ourselves whatever we please?

The word itself provides some interesting leads. In its earliest English usage (1813), "biology" did not mean (as it does today) "the science of life," but rather "the study of human life and character." This meaning is faithful to the Greek root, *bios*, which is not "life" as such, nor animate or animal life—for these, the Greeks used *zoe*—but "a course of life" or "a manner of living," "a *human* life as lived," describable in a *bio*-graphy. When the term "biology" entered the English language, the study of what is now covered by biology was divided between phycology (1658) or botany (1696) and zoology (1669), the study, respectively, of plants and animals. Or else it was conducted under the singular rubric of physiology, the *logos* of *phusis,* a term which at first meant the study of nature (*phusis*) altogether (1564), but soon (1615) became "the science of normal function and phenomena of living things," those beings held to be paradigmatically natural because they sprout (*phuein*), come to birth (*natus sum*), come into being and pass away—on their own, regularly, recurrently.

The point of this etymologizing is to frame the following questions: Does biology today, defined as the science of *life,* do justice to the *beings* that live, to the plants and animals that come to be and pass away, one by one, and that reproduce themselves after their kind? What happens to our understanding of life once science evicts living beings from the center of the natural world; once they come to be understood largely through the concepts of modern physics (and chemistry), which studies nature regarded fundamentally as dead matter-in-motion? Does biology today, as the science of life, do justice to *human* life, which is always lived in formed lives, *bioi,* shaped not only by genetics and physiology but by human aspirations, choices and beliefs, and by cultural institutions, practices and norms? Does biology—*can* biology—teach us anything important about the *nature* of human life or the manner in which it might best be lived?

My conclusion can be simply stated in advance: there are indeed profound and permanent incapacities and restrictions of biology. Moreover, these incapacities follow directly from biology's defects precisely in the matter of limits or boundaries: (1) in modern practice, it foolishly pursues limitless goals; (2) in modern theory, it proceeds by methods and concepts that impose artificial boundaries that are not true to life; and (3) at any time, it faces insuperable limitations posed both by the deficiencies of human reason and by the mysteries of its subject, life itself.

## Practical Limitations:
## The Limitations of Limitless Goals

Though it is commonplace to distinguish *applied* from *pure* science—and it makes some sense to do so—it is important to grasp the essentially practical, social and technical character of modern science as such, modern biology included. Ancient biology had sought knowledge of *what living things are,* to be contemplated as an end in itself, satisfying to the knower. In contrast, modern biology seeks knowledge of *how they work,* to be used as a means for the relief and comfort of all humanity, knowers and non-knowers alike. Though the benefits were at first slow in coming, this practical intention has been at the heart of all of modern science right from the start. In order to make thought useful for meeting human needs, Descartes (in his *Discourse on Method*) proposed a new kind of thinking. He permanently turned his—and science's—back on the speculative or theoretical questions, questions about the being or nature or goodness of things, questions also about first or ultimate causes. Instead, in order to become practical, science will study nature-at-work, nature-as-craftsman; a new kind of physics, solving problems about force and action, will yield power and will ultimately lead to human mastery and ownership of nature.

The purposes of a science-based mastery are humanitarian, served by a boundless medicine capable of curing "an infinitude of maladies both of body and mind," capable perhaps of conquering aging, and even mortality itself. Moreover, because the new medicine will know precisely the mind's dependence on the disposition of the bodily organs, it will be able to provide psychic peace and new mental powers, including a new kind of practical wisdom. *Physics,* here meaning "natural science," will issue in *mastery* of nature (*phusis*), via a new *physick,* an omnicompetent and comprehensive medicine of body and mind.

Descartes' prophecy began to be realized only in our century, and especially for biology and medicine, in the last fifty years. We are showered on all sides by benefits from biomedical technology, including prevention and cures for diseases of mind and body, and considerable increases in overall life expectancy. But though we expect many more benefits yet to come, we are learning, painfully, that these benefits are not unmixed. We are beginning to notice that power over nature is power that can be restricted and withheld from some, misused and abused by others; that even the benevolent uses of humanitarian technologies often have serious unintended and undesired consequences; that as old diseases are conquered, new and often worse ones spring up to take their place; that longer life does not necessarily mean better life; that the ability to intervene technologically in the human body and mind brings vexing dilemmas, anxious fears and sorrowful consequences—about abortion, genetic manipulation, organ transplantation, euthanasia, and use and abuse of drugs; and, worst of all, that the conquest of nature for the relief of man's estate could lead to severe dehumanization— in C. S. Lewis's words, to "the abolition of man."[1] We learn to prevent all genetic disease, but only by turning procreation into manufacture. We have safe and shame-free sex, but little romance or lasting intimacy. We find a perfect "soma" that can cure depression and relieve anxiety, but its unpreventable spread produces people who know and want only chemically induced satisfactions. We live much longer, but can't remember why we wanted to.

The new biology that brings us these dilemmas can, by its very value-neutral self-definition, provide us neither knowledge nor guidance for dealing with them. Worse, the scientific teachings themselves challenge and embarrass the existing prescientific or religious notions of better and worse, and of human life more generally, on the basis of which we have made—and still make—moral judgments; on the basis of which we have lived—and still live—our lives. The project for the mastery of nature, even as it provides limitless powers, leaves the "master" lost at sea. Lacking knowledge of ends and goals, lacking standards of good and bad, right and wrong, we know not who we are nor where we are going. Yet we travel fast and freely, progressively achieving our own estrangement—from our communities, from our nature, from our very selves.

Despite these obvious practical and moral threats to our humanity, scientists and others often refuse to recognize the danger, and even object to the term "dehumanization." For how, they ask, can science or technology be dehumanizing when these activities are themselves the expression of our highest humanity—of our curiosity and courage, our cleverness and dexterity, our energy and industry, our rationality and perfectibility? But not everything of human *origin* is humanizing in *effect*. Man does not live by rationality alone. Indeed, the foundations of our humanity—our sentiments, loves, attitudes, mores and character, as well as the familial, social, religious and political institutions that nourish and are nourished by them—are not laid by scientific reason or rational technique, and may, in truth, be undermined by them, especially if our much-vaunted scientific rationality is—as I hope next to show—philosophically unsound and finally unreasonable.

## Philosophical Limitations: Lifeless Concepts

I have abbreviated my treatment of the practical limitations of biology, partly because they are better known and because they are treated in the previous chapters, but mainly to concentrate instead on the *philosophical* limitations, which are, I believe, less recognized yet also more profound. We can perhaps adjust to our Brave New Worldly biomedical technologies; we may even be able to muddle through without clear and well-grounded moral notions of better and worse. But we will still face, in mind and in spirit, the disquieting disjunction between the vibrant living world we inhabit and enjoy as human beings, and the limited, artificial, lifeless, objectified re-presentation of that world as we learn it from modern biology.

The disjunction between the world-as-experienced and the world-as-known-by-science is, of course, an old story. For example, according to obvious experience a table is hard and solid, but according to atomic physics it is mainly empty space. Most of us say, "so what?" About rocks and tables, this discrepancy is rarely bothersome. But when it reaches to life and to our *human* lives, it is—and will be—increasingly disorienting, troubling, self-alienating.

We need not look far to discover why our biological concepts and approaches are so divorced from life as lived. The divorce was produced deliberately, knowingly, and for a reason. For the adoption of the objectified view of nature (and life) is intimately connected with, and indispensable for, the practical goals of the new science.

To conquer nature-in-its-ordinary-course, we had to find and follow the regularities of a hidden nature reconceived beyond experience. People generally believe that the new science taught us how to find the truth about nature, in the firm hope that solid knowledge would then be useful: Seek knowledge, and knowledge will give you power. But as Richard Kennington has powerfully argued,[2] it would be more accurate to say that the new science sought *first* power over nature, and *derivatively* found a way to reconceive nature that yielded the empowering kind of knowledge: Seek power, and you will be able to devise a way of knowing that gives it to you. The result can be simply put: knowledge permitting prediction and (some) control over biological *events* has been purchased at the cost of deep ignorance, not to say misunderstanding, of *living beings,* ourselves included. It is these limitations—permanently inherent in our reigning biology—that I would now like to clarify.

The first theoretic limitation of modern biology is, ironically, its blindness to the importance of natural boundaries or distinctions. Let us call this distorting tendency *homogenization,* a tendency implicit already in the notion that biology is a universal science of "life." I put quotation marks around this word because it is an abstraction; what lives are individual plants and animals. Moreover, each living individual is a particular one of some specific kind. The differing visible "looks" announce, so to speak, the differences among the various kinds; indeed, within certain species, the looks reveal *individual* differences, as well as different *stages* of the life cycle and different *hierarchical* ranks within a social group. These distinctive "looks," we suspect, reflect distinctive ways of being alive and experiencing life.[3]

Yet virtually all of modern biology abstracts from the manifest heterogeneity of living beings, and instead studies vital processes considered homogeneously. Specific organisms are, of course, selected for study, but they are examined not for their own sake but because they are especially suitable and useful for, say, the search for the universal genetic code and its translation, or the uniform mechanisms of natural selection and speciation, or the universal biochemical processes of metabolism and energy transfer. Largely indifferent to differences in ways of life, biology declares all beings to be in the same business—survival, adaptation, reproduction. Varieties of form and activity are thought not to be revealing and are finally deemed unimportant. But is all this homogeneity true to life?

Homogenization of form, individuality and rank is tied to the second distorting tendency, *analysis and reduction.* Whole organisms are confusing; it is easier to study their parts. Even the visible parts are too confusing. For greater precision, one works with cells or cell-free systems or, ideally, with isolated and purified molecules. Organisms are explained in terms of genes; vital functions are "explained" by the motions and interactions of nonliving molecules. This is, up to a point, a perfectly reasonable strategy; but we must not forget that we are getting a *partial*—both biased and incomplete—view. The functions of the "parts" (for example, the genes and the proteins) studied in isolation often differ from what they are normally, that is, when they are, indeed, parts of the whole. Further, the wholes have powers and activities not found in the parts alone. Why, even the very existence of the whole *as a whole* is inexplicable on reductionist grounds. What accounts for the special unity and active wholeness of each living being, and the effort it makes, instinctively, to preserve its integrity? Analysis will never be able to say.

Drunk on the success of biochemical analysis and molecular genetics, some scientists are predicting, for example, that human love will soon have a chemical explanation. Biologists will isolate that putative small molecule, located in the hypothalamus, whose concentration soars when someone falls in love. Or, again, the national campaign to sequence the entire human genome is virtually complete, and we are told that knowing the chemical sequence will reveal the "secret" of human life. Extreme reductionists go still further. They not only explain the being and workings of wholes in terms of parts; they claim that the whole exists only to serve the parts. They hold, for example, that the real secret of life is that life serves the genes, that all the activities of a differentiated organism are really in the service of turning one genome into two—that the chicken is just an egg's—or its genes'—way of making more eggs or genes.

But is this true to life as lived? These reductionists speak loosely and not well: they mistake knowledge of the part for truth about the whole. Even if a peptide is found that, when injected into the brain, stimulates something like the sensation of falling in love, would that really be an *explanation* of love? Would anyone who ever loved accept, as adequate to the phenomenon, that love *is* (nothing but) an elevated concentration of "erotogenin" in the blood?

Reduction is all the more misleading because of the third distorting tendency, *materialism,* the prejudice that seeks to explain the structure and activity of organized bodies solely in terms of their materials. For example, the activity of transporting substances across cell boundaries is explained by specific transport proteins located in the cell surface; or, again, sight is explained by light-absorbing pigments located in the retina. True, the proteins and the pigments are indispensable, but their physiological function depends also on their placement and integration into larger organized units—the cell membrane, or the eye and visual nervous system. Not the materials as such, but the materials as *organized* are efficacious—and the organization or form is, by definition, *immaterial.* Further, organization of simpler materials makes possible properties and powers not found in the materials alone; the light-absorbing chemicals do not *see* the light they absorb. And powers—capacities for activity—are not themselves material, even though they "reside in" and are inseparable from material. Aristotle made the point ages ago: an organ—for example, the eye—has magnitude, has extension, takes up space; you can hold the eye (or the brain) in your hand. But the *power of sight*—or the *activity of seeing*—has neither magnitude nor extension; one cannot touch or hold or point to "sight."[4] A blind neuroscientist could give precise quantitative details regarding electrical discharges in the eye produced by the stimulus of light, and a blind craftsman could with instruction build a good material model of the eye; but sight can be known only by one who sees. Is it true to life to identify it solely with its material substratum?

Modern biology is not only materialistic but also *mechanistic;* indeed, it delights in nothing so much as working out "the mechanism of action" of innumerable vital phenomena. Not "what is it?" or "what is it for?" but "how does it work?" is the basic question. The mechanical model in modern biology goes back at least to Descartes. In the *Discourse on Method,* Descartes treats all vital activity of animals and all human activity, except for speech and will, in terms of heat and local motion: not only the life-giving motion of the heart and blood, but also wakefulness and sleep, sensing, remembering, imagining, suffering passions, and many bodily motions—all these are at bottom just different forms of local motion. And all motion, including vital motion, is understood mechanically, like the motion of a clock or automaton.

Descartes does not say the organism is, in fact, a machine, but that we do well to *consider* it as a machine—for the sake of certain and useful knowledge (know-how). But is this mechanical account—or any mechanical account—sufficient, even for these limited purposes? Granted, vital processes occur in an orderly way, but does that make them fundamentally mechanical? The mechanical account leaves no room for spontaneity or self-initiated action. It ignores all inwardness of the agent: interested awareness, felt lack, appetite, intentionality and, hence, the purposiveness of lived movement—all are ignored. However useful as a heuristic concept, the mechanical account is not true to life.

The emphasis on mechanism is an expression of the *nonteleological* character of modern biology, a fifth feature not true to life. As I have argued elsewhere,[5] living things must be regarded as purposive beings, as beings that cannot even be looked at, much less properly described or fully understood, without teleological notions. Organisms come-into-being through an orderly, self-directed process of differentiation that reaches an internally determined end or completion. At each stage, but most fully when mature, each is an organic and active whole, a unity of structure and function, the parts contributing to the maintenance and working of the whole. Wholeness is preserved through remarkable powers of self-healing, each organism acting unconsciously from within to restore its own integrity—which it somehow both "knows" and "wants." Other characteristic activities of each organism stretch above and beyond mere self-maintenance. Living things display directedness, inner "striving" toward a goal, activities that transcend confinement to the here and now:

> A seedling sprouting beneath a large rock will bend and grow around the rock to reach the light. A young bird will continue to struggle to coordinate wing and tail motions until it finally learns to fly. A beaver will make many trips to build a dam, or a bird a nest, or a spider a web.... And for many animals there is an elaborate pattern of behavior leading up to mating. *In none of these cases is the activity planned or conscious or intended, yet it is just the same a directed and inwardly determined activity to an end for a purpose.*[6]

To be sure, one can study the *how* of these activities mechanistically; but one ought not conclude therefrom that purposiveness is an illusion.

Some biologists are quite willing to admit purpose into biology, but only in the case of human beings. Because they believe there can be no purposive behavior without conscious intention or choice, they deny purposiveness to animals but allow it for themselves. (A good thing, too; otherwise, their own purposive and goal-directed behavior as biologists would refute them.) For these scientists, the mechanistic outlook of modern biology leads to a dualistic view of man—a view expressed even among some leading neurophysiologists who now concede that consciousness and free will cannot be reduced to or explained by the physiological mechanics of the brain. They have returned to something like the basic dualism of Descartes: man, alone among living things, has "soul," or a principle of "reason-will-consciousness," but in other respects he can be understood mechanistically, like other plants and animals.

The relation of this "mind-soul" to the soulless body machine— the so-called mind-body problem—remains an embarrassment for materialists and mechanists, and it is premature to guess how future biological findings may change the shape of the debate. But we notice, with suspicion, two problematic implications: First, the mind-body dualism unreasonably sunders consciousness from bodily life. Much of that of which we become conscious penetrates "upward" from "below"; the unimpeded, unconscious activity of the living-body-inaction—say, in dancing—lights up the soul with feelings of pleasure. Conversely, psychosomatic interactions going the other way—such as the involuntary blush of conscious embarrassment—also cast doubt on any assertion of strict dualism. Second, the theory of evolution, connecting man to the rest of animate nature, casts doubt both on the dualistic account of man, and also on the adequacy of mechanism for understanding the rest of life. Either man, too—his felt sense of inwardness, freedom, mind, consciousness and purposiveness notwithstanding—is to be assimilated to the blind and dumb world of mechanism, or the rest of living nature must again be seen more in the light of what common sense has always taken to be naturally and purposefully human. Though no major philosopher since Descartes has attributed soul to animals and plants, these reflections would reopen the possibility that "soul"—and inwardness and purposiveness—is, in truth, found everywhere among the living.[7]

The subject of evolution prompts one or two brief observations, merely in passing, for evolutionary biology has limitations of its own. Though there is today a growing debate about the mechanisms of evolution, the reigning orthodoxy still credits accidental mutation and natural selection as the major means of evolutionary change. Yet very few people have noticed that this nonteleological explanation of change not only assumes but even depends upon the immanent teleological character of all living organisms. The desire or tendency of living things to stay alive and their endeavor to reproduce, both of which are among the minimal conditions of Darwinian theory, are taken for granted and unexplained. It is only part of an explanation to say that those beings with no tendency to maintain and reproduce themselves have died out. Why are the other ones, the self-maintaining and reproducing beings, here at all? They are not teleological *because* they have survived; on the contrary, they have survived (in part) because they are teleological. Can evolutionary biology tell us why a nonteleological nature would generate and sustain teleological beings? Or why, over time, it would give rise to higher organisms, with a fuller range of powers of awareness, desire and action? Do we really understand what we are claiming when we accept the view that a mindless universe gave rise to mind? One begins to wonder whether permanence, stability and perpetuation exhaust the goals of living things. As Whitehead put it:

In fact life itself is comparatively deficient in survival value. The art of persistence is to be dead. ... A rock survives for eight hundred million years; whereas the limit for a tree is about a thousand years, for a man or an elephant about fifty or one hundred years, for a dog about twelve years, for an insect about one year. The problem set by the doctrine of evolution is to explain how complex organisms with such deficient survival power ever evolved.[8]

Our current evolutionary orthodoxy has, in fact, little to say about the true origin of life or about ultimate causes, not only of life but of all major biological novelty. It cannot account for the emergence of higher organisms, who often seem more engaged with mediated activity than with the necessities of survival and reproduction; think, for example, of the play of kittens and monkeys or the frolicking of otters and sea lions. Orthodoxy requires us to believe that these free and enjoyable activities must be *useful,* must have some selective advantage in the struggle to survive or to leave more progeny. Tyrannically rejecting all other explanations of change, the theory of natural selection sometimes even blinds us to the existence of certain phenomena that would be very difficult to attribute to natural selection (for example, the descent of the testes in mammals); we learn to see only what orthodoxy can explain. If its favorite theory constricts our vision, how can modern biology present a full view of life?

But there remains one special feature of modern biology, itself a cardinal premise of modern science altogether, that seems to be both most powerful in yielding new knowledge of biological events and, at the same time, *most* untrue to life: the principle of *objectification.* Because of its centrality, I shall treat it at somewhat greater length.

The term "objective" has both a common colloquial meaning and a precise philosophical meaning, the former descending from the latter but without our knowing what distortions we have swallowed in the process. In common speech, we are inclined to use "objective" as a synonym for "true" or "real." Not only a scientist but any fair-minded person is supposed "to be objective": unprejudiced, disinterested, rational, free from contamination of merely personal—that is, subjective—bias or perspective, and able therefore to capture so-called "objective reality." "Objective reality" is the domain especially of the sciences, because the methodical pursuit of reproducible and shareable findings guarantees their objective status.

This common view is, in fact, somewhat misleading, for it is a mistake to regard "the objective" as synonymous with "the true" or "the real." Pursuit of the error discloses, surprisingly, an unbridgeable gap between science and reality, and, in our case, between the science of biology and the living nature it studies. *For the so-called objective view of nature is not nature's own, but one imposed on nature, imposed by none other than the interested human subject.*

Here's how this works. An "object," literally, means that which is "thrown-out-before-and-against" us—thrown by, thrown-before-and-against, and existing for and relative to the human subject who "did the throwing." Not the natural world, *but the self-thinking human subject,* is the source of objectivity. The interested subject's demand for clear and distinct and certain "knowledge" leads him to *re*-present the given world before his mind, in an act of deliberate projection, through concepts (invented for the purpose) that allow him to operate mentally on the world with utmost (usually quantitative) precision. What cannot be grasped through such conceptual re-presentation drops from view. Only those aspects of the world that can be "objectified" (or quantified) become objects for scientific study. The given, visible and tangible world of our experience is banished into the shadows; the shadowy world of "concepts" gains the limelight and reconfigures everything in sight, giving them an "objectified" character that is at best only partially true to what they *are.*

The classic example of this objectification of the world has in fact to do with the world as visible and, by implication, with ourselves as viewers. In a revolution-making passage in the *Rules for the Direction of the Mind,* Descartes sets the program for all of modern science by radically transforming how we should approach the study of color:

> Thus whatever you suppose color *to be,* you cannot deny *that it is extended* and in consequence possessed of figure. Is there then any *disadvantage,* if, while taking care not to admit any new entity uselessly, or rashly to imagine that it exists ... but merely abstracting from every other feature except that it

possesses the nature of figure, we conceive the diversity existing between white, blue, and red, etc., as being like the difference between the following similar figures?

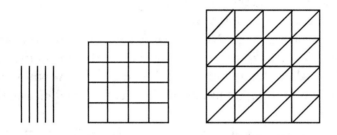

The same argument applies to all cases; for it is certain that the *infinitude of figures* suffices to *express* all the differences in sensible things.[9] [Emphasis added.]

To see more clearly what is involved in "objectification" and how it distorts the very phenomena in the course of coming to "understand" them, let us go slowly through the passage, noting the following crucial points:

1. We are told to ignore the *being* or *nature* of color, and concentrate instead only on the "fact" that, because colored *things* are extended (that is, take up space), all *color* has figure or shape. ("Never mind," say Descartes, "what color really *is*. You cannot deny that *it* has figure.")*

2. We then must *abstract* from every feature of color *except* that it has the nature of *figure*. Why? For an advantage in knowing, yet a kind of knowing that is indifferent to existence, to what something really *is*. The knowledge acquired by objectification is indifferent or neutral to the *being* or *reality* of things.

---

*Compare the relation of color and shape *(schema)* suggested by Socrates in Plato's *Meno:* "Shape is that which, alone among all things, always accompanies color." (75B6) Appealing to our primary experience of the visible world, this account integrates shape and color as the two most evident and always related aspects of any visible body, whose shaped surface we come to see only because of color differences between it and its surroundings. To put it crudely, Socrates' philosophizing deepens lived experience; Descartes' turns its back on lived experience.

3. The act of this reconception is a willful act of mind. Descartes *decides* or *chooses* to conceive the truth about color under the concept of figure. We do not, as knowers, try to catch the *natural* looks of *visible things;* instead, by decision, *we choose* to *conceive* (literally, "to grasp together") or represent before our grasping minds only *certain* aspects of the world.

4. Which aspects? Not the natures of colors, not the being of colors, but the *differences* among them ("the *diversity* existing between white, blue, and red"). We do not seek to know *things* through and through, but only their external—and measurable— *relations.*

5. The *natural* differences are "translated"—or, rather, *symbolized*—by *mathematical* ones. The differences of color are represented by differences among similar figures. Why? Because if we con-figure things, we can then take their mathematical measure, using the radically new mathematics of quantity (featuring the number line and analytic geometry) that Descartes has invented for this purpose, a mathematics that introduced terms of arithmetic (traditionally the study of *discrete* multitudes) into the study of geometry (the study of *continuous* magnitudes). The analytic geometry of Cartesian space is the perfect vehicle for precise measurement of anything—space, time, mass, density, volume, velocity, energy, temperature, blood pressure, drunkenness, intelligence or scholastic achievement that can be treated as an extent or quantity or dimension.

6. Descartes' geometrical figures may be poor and passé as standing for the differences among the colors white, blue and red, but the principle he proposes is not: today we still treat color in terms of "wavelengths," purely mathematical representations *from which all the color is sucked out.* This tells the whole story: *the objective is purely quantitative. All quality disappears.*

7. Objectification can be universalized: says Descartes, *all the differences* (that is, changes or relations) in sensible things—that is, in every being that exists in the natural world—can be expressed mathematically. The world—or more accurately, *changes* in the world—can be represented objectively, as differences among figures (or, eventually, in equations). The multifaceted and profound world of things is replaced by a shadowy network of mathematized relations. Objectified knowledge is ghostly, to say the least.

In this classic example, we have the touchstone of all so-called objective knowledge. The objectified world is, by deliberate design, abstract, purely quantitative, homogeneous, and indifferent to the question of being or existence. "Things" are "known" only externally and relationally. Moreover, the symbolic representations used to handle the objectified world bear absolutely no relation to the thing represented: a wavelength or a mathematical equation neither resembles nor points to color.

No one gets very excited about the objectification of color, but we become suspicious when science tries to objectify the *viewing* of color or, worse, the *viewer*. And now we see why. By its very principle, "objective knowledge" of sight and seeing will not be—because it *cannot* be—true to lived experience; for lived experience is always qualitative, concrete, heterogeneous, suffused with the attention, interest and engaged concern of the living soul. Real seeing can never be captured by wavelengths, absorption spectra of retinal cells, or electrical depolarizations and discharges in the objectified brain. Likewise also the inwardness of life, including awareness, appetite, emotion, and the genuine and interested relations between one living being and others, both friend and foe; or the engaged, forward-pointed, outward-moving tendencies of living beings; or the uniqueness of each individual life as lived in living time, from birth to death; the concern of each animal (conscious or not) for its own health, wholeness and well-being—none of these essential aspects of nature alive fall within the cramped and distorting boundaries of nature objectified.

Honesty compels me to interrupt this critique and tell you one last and, indeed, astounding part of this tale, one which, I suspect, you already know. Objectification works! For some reason, the many-splendored world of nature allows itself to be grasped by the anemic concepts of objective science. Never mind that it is partial, distorted, shadowy, abstract; the quantitative approach has put men on the moon, lights on the ceiling, and pacemakers in our hearts. Somehow, it must be capturing well at least one aspect of being. It is, to speak unscientifically, a miracle!

To sum up this major part of the argument: modern biology has carefully defined its conceptual and methical boundaries in such a way that it is inherently incapable of understanding life as lived—not only by human beings, but by any living being. It is inherently incapable of understanding that (and why) living beings are ordered and active wholes, particular ones of a particular kind; individually unique, time-bound, and experiencing a nuanced journey between birth and death; perishable and needy and, therefore, aspiring and energetically self-concerned. It is incapable of understanding that (and why) living beings are self-developing, self-maintaining, self-moving beings, each with a relation to its own world, mediated always by "inwardness," however rudimentary, comprising awareness of and appetition for things beyond their boundaries. It is incapable of understanding that (and why) they are purposive, serving both themselves and their descendants; that (and why) their patterned surfaces are on display, often revealing—in part—various communicable aspects of the state of the soul within; that (and how, and why) there is a hierarchy of capacities and powers—within a given life, within social groupings of the same species, and in the entire kingdom of living things overall. True, our biology promises and can deliver a limitless string of intriguing and useful discoveries, within the boundaries it has set for itself, about many diverse vital phenomena. But the nature and meaning of living beings, and of life altogether, will forever lie out of reach. Modern biology will never be able to tell us what life *is*, what is *responsible* for it, or what it is *for*. It will never be able to say, about even the simplest plant or animal, what it is, what its life is truly like, or what its flourishing or well-being might be.

## Alternative Biologies: Ultimate Limits

To be fair, I must now confess that not all of modern biology adheres fully to the orthodox view I have presented and whose limits I have tried to show. Recently, there have been increasing objections to reductionism, with new suggestions that each "level of organization"—that is, molecules, organelles, cells, tissues, organs, organisms, social groupings, and such—must be treated on its own terms. There are challenges to the sufficiency of materialism, at least with respect to explaining the human mind and consciousness. In evolutionary theory, there is opposition to the orthodox view that all evolutionary novelty is the result of small and accidental random mutations, and some people are flirting with suggestions (vaguely Lamarckian) that lived experience can effect changes in heritable genotype. Yet though welcome, none of these challenges are likely to burst through the conceptual barrier, precisely because they accept the "objectified" view of the world on which modern biology is grounded.

But there are unorthodox biologists, some of them contemporary, who present truly alternative approaches to life. For example, there is the late Adolf Portmann, who did remarkable studies on the communicative and aesthetic meaning of animal appearance, and its relation to genuine social life;[10] the late Erwin Straus, who developed a rich phenomenological psychology and a nonobjectified understanding of sensing;[11] Oliver Sacks, who has emphasized the acquired individuation of each "nervous system";[12] E. S. Russell, who explored the purposive directedness of vital activities;[13] and (the philosopher) Hans Jonas, who has elaborated a coherent and hierarchic account of life around the notion of "needful freedom," held always precariously in the face of the threat of extinction.[14] Recently making a comeback among students of natural philosophy, there is Goethe, a connoisseur of morphology who, well before Darwin, explored the immanent creative powers of life and who understood, perhaps better than anyone else, how the purposive yet innovative mind of man might both mirror and embody the purposiveness and creativity of nature itself.[15] And hiding off-stage, but still accessible to us, is that first biologist of nature-in-its-ordinary-course, Aristotle, who emphasized questions of being over becoming, form over matter, purposiveness over moving causes, and wholes over parts; for whom the soul was not an ethereal spirit or a ghost-in-the-machine but an immanent and embodied principle of all vital activity; and for whom science was a refined and ever-deepening reflection on the natures and the causes of the beings manifest to us in ordinary experience, requiring neither abdication of our human point of view, nor an artificial reconception of the world, nor the neglect of phenomena that theory cannot explain.[16] These all commend themselves to our attention, at least for their questions and concerns, if we are interested in enlarging the boundaries and reducing the limitations of a richer biology closer to its living subject. Yet

I wish to insist that there may be permanent limitations for the study of life, even for the most natural of biologies—even for a biology that again learned to speak of living form or *telos* or soul. There are at least four limitations that may well be insurmountable, two having to do with the limitations of speech and reason, two having to do with the enigmas of our subject.

First, study, as such, dissolves the unity of the living being. Although soul-and-body or form-and-matter are, in being, concrete, grown-together, and as inseparable as the concave and the convex, speech divides them and cannot bespeak their true unity. The point was made already by Aristotle. What, he asks, is anger? The dialecticians say it is the desire for revenge, to give pain for slight; the physiologists say it is a warming of the blood around the heart. Who is right? Answer: Both together.[17] But not even Aristotle, the master of *logos,* can speak them truly together; he can speak them only side by side. Aristotle, for all his hylomorphism and talk of psychosomatic unity, has as much trouble as we do restoring unity once the dissection of discursive speech begins.

Second, science as such abstracts and homogenizes. Science seeks generalizations, living beings are particular. How can even the most natural of biologies do justice to the ineffability of individuality if science, by definition, is about the necessary and the universal, while individuality, though real, is contingent and particular? Science, as the search for causes, tends to abstract from real differences, not only among individuals but even among species. This question, too, already troubled Aristotle. He knew that each species had a separate nature or *eidos*—lions give birth only to lions, and porcupines only to porcupines; and this suggests that science—knowledge of the separate *natures* of things—should proceed species by species. Yet because explaining the functioning of the parts of animals would require him repetitiously to say much the same thing about all similar higher animals, he (reluctantly, it seems) took a more generalizing approach.[18] And when he came, in *De Anima,* to the discussion of the powers of the soul, it turned out that there were really only three or four basic soul types—the vegetative soul, the (proto)sensitive soul and (its higher form) the appetitive soul, and the rational soul. From the viewpoint of "souling"—that is, the activities of nourishing, sensing, desiring—panthers and leopards and cheetahs and tigers and lions are roughly equivalent. The *science* of life always violates life's living particularity.

Third, life and soul are irreducibly mysterious. Science, whether objective or natural (modern or premodern), seeks to clarify what is obscure, seeks to explain what is perplexing or wondrous. Today's science is overconfident of its ability to do so; it treats "mystery" as simply that which has not *yet* been understood. To insist, today, that nature contains *real* mysteries—things *incapable* of being understood—is generally to plead guilty to scientific heresy; for this, one gets called a mystic and is encouraged to transfer to the theology department. Yet the greatest scientists have sometimes openly confessed their sense not only of wonder but also of awe, as they confronted phenomena that defy full capture by reason. In all times and places, the biologist confronted with living beings has privileged access to the truly awesome and mysterious: the emergence of a new life, never seen before; the extinction of a life in death, lost and gone forever; the question of how life first emerged, and why; the enormous possibilities for existences different from his own, manifest in nature's prodigality throughout the living world; and, mystery of mysteries, the nature of his own soul—entwined with his body, here and now, as the integrated powers of his perishable life; and yet sufficiently free from the constraints of body, place and time to freely biologize, to think any thought, receive any idea, be transported in mind to faraway times and places, contemplate truly timeless truths. If he allowed himself to wonder at his own mindful life, a truly open biologist would be brought to the brink of the unfathomable: Can the same "thing" be both cause of life or change and cause of awareness? How, indeed, if the soul is that which moves (us), can it also be that which knows?*

Finally, there is the insufficiency of nature for ethics. This last observation points up the difficulty in looking to biology—even to

---

*This is the ancient conundrum about the soul. It informs the discussion of the soul in Plato's *Phaedo*, and probably accounts for the unavoidably inconclusive character of the argument for the soul's immortality. Jacob Klein has pointed out that never does the famous Socratic "What is" question get raised about the soul, though all the dialogues are somehow about the soul. According to Klein, this suggests that, for Plato, the soul is *not* an *eidos*, not a simple or single *idea* or thing.

a more natural science more true to life—for very much help in answering the questions about how we are to live. It is, to be frank, a path worth following, and I myself have been pursuing it for nearly thirty years. The hope can be simply stated: if we really understood human nature and human wholeness, we would be better able to discern human flourishing and the human good. A noble aspiration—and not utterly fruitless.[19] But there are obvious difficulties, especially if the human being turns out not to be simple, that is, turns out to have more than one good or *telos*—as, it seems, he clearly does. Why, even among the animals, there is a tension between self-love (or self-preservation) and the urge to reproduce. To reproduce means voting with your feet for your own demise. To be a sexual being is to be self-divided and incomplete—as we learn from the story of Adam and Eve, whose discovery of their nakedness was the first insight of an awakened human self-consciousness. Worse, for the thinking animal, the very desire for knowledge is, in principle, at odds with the demands of life. In truth, the loves of life, especially human life, do not sing the same song. True, a richer biology might clarify what these longings really seek. It might contribute to a richer understanding of a healthy soul. But the task of harmonizing competing goods, both for any individual and especially *among* individuals who seek them variously, will always remain the work of a largely autonomous ethical and political science, helped, where possible, with insights mysteriously received from sources not under strict human command. Biology may do some of its finest work when it is brought to acknowledge and affirm the mysteries of the soul and the mysterious source of life, truth and goodness.

# Acknowledgments

Thanks are owed to many people who helped me produce this volume. Irving Kristol, Adam Wolfson, Neal Kozodoy, Leon Wieseltier and Jim Nuechterlein, fine editors all, improved the original versions of the essays. My good friends Irving and Bea Kristol urged me a year and a half ago to collect my essays into a single volume. Yuval Levin, my former student and now colleague, read through all the essays, offering valuable editorial advice and suggesting a logical order for the volume that guided my rewriting. My son-in-law Robert Hochman helped me analyze the Supreme Court decisions in the "right to die" cases. Peter Collier, editor, publisher and gracious guide, eagerly embraced this project at Encounter Books and offered astute editorial suggestions that I was only too pleased to follow. I am deeply grateful to Christopher DeMuth and to Roger and Susan Hertog for the position they have made available to me at the American Enterprise Institute, where this project was brought to completion.

I dedicate this volume to three friends and mentors: Harvey Flaumenhaft, dean of St. John's College in Annapolis, closest friend, and interlocutor for nearly half a century, who helped cure me of my youthful utopianism and who introduced me to the fundamental books and ideas that have guided my search for an alternative; the late Hans Jonas, whose moral passion and philosophical courage inspired me and whose friendship encouraged me; and the late Paul Ramsey, my first guide in biomedical ethics, whose principled devotion to moral clarity and sound reasoning remains for me a beacon in an age in which even bioethicists are now for sale.

As always, my deepest gratitude, inexpressible, is to Amy.

# Notes

## Introduction

[1] "Babies by Means of in vitro Fertilization: Unethical Experiments on the Unborn?" *New England Journal of Medicine* 285 (1971): 1174–79; "Making Babies—the New Biology and the 'Old' Morality," *Public Interest*, Winter 1972; and "'Making Babies' Revisited," *Public Interest*, Winter 1979. For a general overview of my earlier thoughts on bioethical matters, see *Toward a More Natural Science: Biology and Human Affairs* (New York: The Free Press, 1985; paperback, 1988).

## Chapter 1: The Problem of Technology and Liberal Democracy

[1] See, for example, Plato's *Gorgias* 450C.

[2] Aristotle, *Nicomachean Ethics* 1140a20.

[3] Martin Heidegger, "The Question Concerning Technology," in *The Question Concerning Technology and Other Essays*, trans. William Lovitt (New York: Harper & Row, 1977), esp. pp. 14–17.

[4] Jacques Ellul, *The Technological Society*, trans. John Wilkinson (New York: Vintage Books, 1964), p. 21.

[5] Aeschylus, *Prometheus Bound*, trans. David Grene, in *Aeschylus II*, The Complete Greek Tragedies, ed. David Grene and Richmond Lattimore (Chicago: University of Chicago Press, 1956), lines 250, 437 ff.

[6] Genesis 3:7.

[7] Genesis 11:1–9. See my essay "What's Wrong with Babel?" in *American Scholar*, vol. 58, no. 1 (Winter 1988–89), pp. 41–60.

[8] Francis Bacon, *The Advancement of Learning*, Book I, and *The Interpretation of Nature*, Proem, in *Selected Writings of Francis Bacon*, ed. Hugh G. Dick (New York: Random House, 1955), p. 193 and pp. 150–54.

[9] Robert Smith Woodbury, "History of Technology," *Encyclopaedia Britannica*, 14h ed. (1973), vol. 21, p. 750. Emphasis added.

[10] René Descartes, *Discourse on Method*, in *The Philosophical Works of Descartes*, vol. 1, ed. Elizabeth S. Haldane and G. R. T. Ross (Cambridge, England: Cambridge University Press, 1981), p. 119.

[11] Hans Jonas, *Philosophical Essays: From Ancient Creed to Technological Man* (Englewood Cliffs, New Jersey: Prentice Hall, 1974), p. 48.

[12] Plato, *Republic* VII, 514A ff.

[13] Descartes, *Discourse on Method*, p. 120.

[14] Hans Jonas, *The Imperative of Responsibility: In Search of an Ethics for the Technological Age* (Chicago: University of Chicago Press, 1984), p. 11.

[15] C. S. Lewis, *The Abolition of Man* (New York: Macmillan, 1965), pp. 69–71.

[16] Ellul, *The Technological Society,* ch. 2, "A Characterology of Technique," pp. 61–147, at p. 99.

[17] "The Twentieth Century—Its Promise and Its Realization," speech delivered at Massachusetts Institute of Technology, 31 March 1949, in *Winston Churchill: His Complete Speeches, 1897–1963,* ed. Robert Rhodes James (New York: Chelsea House, 1983), vol. 7, pp. 341–50, at p. 344.

[18] Lewis, *The Abolition of Man,* pp. 77–80.

[19] Jean-Jacques Rousseau, "Discourse on the Origin and Foundations of Inequality among Men," in *The First and Second Discourses,* ed. Roger Masters (New York: St. Martin's Press, 1964), p. 147.

### Chapter 2: Practicing Ethics: Where's the Action?

[1] In Michael Oakeshott, *Rationalism in Politics* (New York: Basic Books, 1962), pp. 59–79.

[2] Ibid., pp. 61–62.

[3] Ibid., pp. 62–63. Emphasis added.

### Chapter 4: The Age of Genetic Technology Arrives

[1] See, for example, LeRoy Walters, "Human Gene Therapy: Ethics and Public Policy," *Human Gene Therapy* 2 (1991): 115–22.

[2] Hans Jonas, "Biological Engineering—A Preview," in his *Philosophical Essays: From Ancient Creed to Technological Man* (Englewood Cliffs, New Jersey: Prentice Hall, 1974), pp. 141–67, at p. 163. Italics in original.

[3] Ibid., p. 161.

[4] Aeschylus, *Prometheus Bound,* lines 250ff.

[5] C. S. Lewis, *The Abolition of Man* (New York: Macmillan, 1965), pp. 69–71. Italics in original.

[6] Bentley Glass, "Science: Endless Horizons or Golden Age?" *Science* 171 (1971): 23–29, at p. 28.

[7] Howard Kaye, "Anxiety and Genetic Manipulation: A Sociological View," *Perspectives in Biology and Medicine* 41, no. 4 (Summer 1998): 483–90, at p. 488. See also Kaye's book *The Social Meaning of Modern Biology,* 2nd ed. (New Brunswick, New Jersey: Transaction Publishers, 1997).

[8] International Academy of Humanism, "Statement in Defense of Cloning and the Integrity of Scientific Research," 16 May 1997.

[9] Steven Pinker, "A Matter of Soul," Correspondence Section, *Weekly Standard,* 2 February 1998, p. 6.

### Chapter 5: Cloning and the Posthuman Future

[1] "Making Babies—the New Biology and the 'Old' Morality," *Public Interest,* Winter 1972.

### Chapter 6: Organs for Sale? Propriety, Property and the Price of Progress

[1] Lloyd R. Cohen, "Increasing the Supply of Transplant Organs: The Virtues of a Futures Market," *George Washington Law Review* 58, no. 1 (November 1989): 1–51. See also Henry Hansmann, "The Economics and Ethics of Markets for Human Organs," *Journal of Health Politics, Policy and Law* 14, no. 1 (1989): 57–86.

[2] Leon. R. Kass, M.D., *Toward a More Natural Science: Biology and Human Affairs* (New York: The Free Press, 1985).

[3] Erwin Straus, *Phenomenological Psychology* (New York: Basic Books, 1966), pp. 137–65.

[4] Kass, *Toward a More Natural Science,* pp. 280–81, 295–98.

[5] Immanuel Kant, *The Metaphysical Principles of Virtue,* trans. James Ellington (Indianapolis: Bobbs-Merrill, 1964), p. 84.

[6] Ibid.

[7] John Locke, *Second Treatise on Civil Government,* Chapter 5, "Of Property."

[8] See, for example, Aristotle's discussion of money and its central importance in commutative justice, *Nicomachean Ethics* 1133a19–1133b28.

[9] Paul Ramsey, "Giving or Taking Cadaver Organs for Transplant," in *The Patient As Person* (New Haven: Yale University Press, 1970), p. 213.

[10] Willard Gaylin, "Harvesting the Dead," *Harper's* 249 (1492), September 1974. The idea Gaylin presents in lurid detail was presented several years earlier by the late Hans Jonas, one of the deepest thinkers about the meaning of the modern technological project. (See his essay "Against the Stream: Comments on the Definition and Redefinition of Death," republished in Hans Jonas, *Philosophical Essays* (Chicago: University of Chicago Press, 1980).

### Chapter 7: Is There a Right to Die?

[1] John Keown, "Some Reflections on Euthanasia in The Netherlands," in *Euthanasia, Clinical Practice, and the Law,* ed. Luke Gormally (London: Linacre Centre for Health Care Ethics, 1994), pp. 193–218, at p. 209. Keown is citing F. C. B. van Wijmen, *Artsen en het Zelfgekozen Levenseinde* (Doctors and the self-chosen termination of life) (Maastricht: Vaakgroep Gezondheidrecht Rijksuniversiteit Limburg, 1989), p. 24, table 18.

[2] Data are from Paul J. van der Maas, et al., *Euthanasia and Other Medical Decisions Concerning the End of Life* (New York: Elsevier Science Inc., 1992), as reported in John Keown, "Further Reflections on Euthanasia in The Netherlands in the Light of the Remmelink Report

and the Van Der Maas Survey," in *Euthanasia, Clinical Practice, and the Law,* ed. Gormally, pp. 219–40, at p. 224.

[3] Gerrit van der Wal, et al., "Evaluation of the Notification Procedure for Physician-Assisted Death in The Netherlands," *New England Journal of Medicine* 335 (1996): 1706–11.

[4] Herbert Hendin, et al., "Physician-Assisted Suicide and Euthanasia in The Netherlands," *JAMA* 277 (1997): 1720–22. For a fuller and chilling account of the Dutch practice, see Herbert Hendin, *Seduced by Death: Doctors, Patients, and the Dutch Cure* (New York: Norton, 1996).

[5] Harvey C. Mansfield Jr., "The Old Rights and the New: Responsibility vs. Self-Expression," in *Old Rights and New,* ed. Robert A. Licht (Washington: AEI, 1992), pp. 97–98.

[6] Hans Jonas, "The Right to Die," *Hastings Center Report,* August 1978, pp. 31–36, at p. 31.

[7] John Locke, *Second Treatise on Civil Government,* Chapter 2, "Of the State of Nature," par. 6.

[8] Ibid., Chapter 5, "Of Property," par. 27. Emphasis added.

[9] See, for example, Rousseau, *Discourse on the Origin and Foundations of Inequality Among Men,* note 9, especially par. 4 and 5.

[10] Immanuel Kant, *The Metaphysical Principles of Virtue,* trans. James Ellington (Indianapolis: Bobbs-Merrill, 1964), pp. 83–84.

[11] Mansfield, "The Old Rights and the New," p. 104.

[12] 497 U.S. 261 (1990).

[13] 521 U.S. 702 (1997) (*Glucksberg*); 521 U.S. 793 (1997) (*Quill*).

[14] Yale Kamisar, "The Rise and Fall of the 'Right' to Assisted Suicide," in *The Case against Assisted Suicide,* ed. Kathleen Foley, M.D., and Herbert Hendin, M.D. (Baltimore: Johns Hopkins University Press, 2002), pp. 69–93, at p. 85. Kamisar's essay provides an excellent analysis of where we are and where we might be going in "right to die" jurisprudence.

### Chapter 8: Death with Dignity and the Sanctity of Life

[1] "Neither for Love nor Money: Why Doctors Must Not Kill," *Public Interest,* Winter 1989, pp. 25–46. An updated version appears in *The Case against Assisted Suicide,* ed. Kathleen Foley, M.D., and Herbert Hendin, M.D. (Baltimore: Johns Hopkins University Press, 2002).

### Chapter 10: The Permanent Limitations of Biology

[1] C. S. Lewis, *The Abolition of Man* (New York: Macmillan, 1965). See especially Chapter 3.

[2] Richard Kennington, unpublished lecture on Francis Bacon, The Committee on Social Thought, The University of Chicago, 1986.

[3] See Adolf Portmann, *Animal Forms and Patterns,* trans. Hella Czech (London: Faber and Faber, 1964; paperback, New York: Schocken

Books, 1967). See also my "Looking Good: Nature and Nobility," in Leon R. Kass, M.D., *Toward a More Natural Science: Biology and Human Affairs* (New York: The Free Press, 1984).

[4] Aristotle, *De Anima* II, 12, 424a25–29.

[5] Leon R. Kass, M.D., "Teleology, Darwinism and the Place of Man: Beyond Chance and Necessity?" in *Toward a More Natural Science,* Chapter 10.

[6] Ibid., p. 256.

[7] See Leon R. Kass, M.D., *The Hungry Soul: Eating and the Perfecting of Our Nature* (New York: The Free Press, 1994; paperback, with a new forward, Chicago: University of Chicago Press, 1999).

[8] Alfred North Whitehead, *The Function of Reason* (Boston: Beacon Press, 1962), pp. 4–5.

[9] René Descartes, *Rules for the Direction of the Mind,* in *The Philosophical Works of Descartes,* ed. Elizabeth S. Haldane and G. R. T. Ross (Cambridge, England: Cambridge University Press, 1981), p. 37.

[10] Portmann, *Animal Forms and Patterns.* See also *Animals As Social Beings,* trans. Oliver Coburn (New York: Viking Press, 1961).

[11] Erwin Straus, *Phenomenological Psychology* (New York: Basic Books, 1966) and *The Primary World of Senses,* trans. J. Needleman (New York: Free Press of Glencoe, 1968).

[12] Oliver Sacks, *Awakenings* (New York: Dutton, 1987).

[13] E. S. Russell, *The Directiveness of Organic Activities* (Cambridge, England: Cambridge University Press, 1945).

[14] Hans Jonas, *The Phenomenon of Life: Toward a Philosophical Biology* (Chicago: University of Chicago Press, 1982).

[15] J. W. Goethe, *Metamorphosis of Plants* and other essays, in *Goethe's Botanical Writings,* trans. Bertha Mueller (Woodbridge, Connecticut: Ox Bow Press, 1989).

[16] Aristotle, *History of Animals, Parts of Animals, Generation of Animals, Locomotion of Animals, Physics B, De Anima.*

[17] Aristotle, *De Anima* I, 1, 403a25–b17.

[18] Aristotle, *Parts of Animals* I, 1 & 5, 639a16–b5, 645b1–14.

[19] Kass, *Toward a More Natural Science,* Chapter 13.

# Index

CPSIA information can be obtained
at www.ICGtesting.com
Printed in the USA
LVHW080855250619
622280LV00004B/11/P